Healthier Living Naturally™

Health and Wellness Guide

Individual|Small Business|Non-Profit|Corporation

I0426677

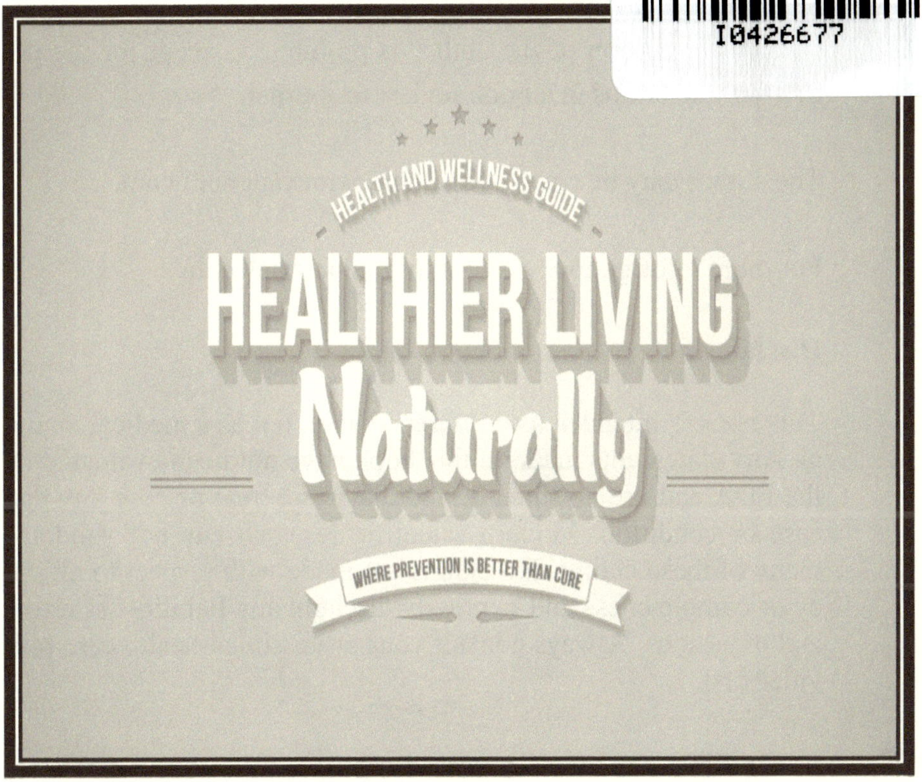

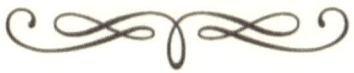

HEALTH AND WELLNESS GUIDE

HEALTHIER LIVING

Naturally

WHERE PREVENTION IS BETTER THAN CURE

CHRISTINA HALL

Healthier Living Naturally™
Health and Wellness Guide

The author may be contacted at hhhjourney@gmail.com.

For more information, go to: http://hhhjourney.com

Disclaimer

This book is dedicated to all those who seek Health, Healing and Hope on this journey we call life.

Contents

Foreword

You may be reading this *Healthier Living Naturally: Health and Wellness Guide* to help you find your way to better health or maybe you've just lost hope and you don't know what else to do. Let me just say that there is ALWAYS hope! My personal health journey started when my own loved one became sick. I decided to seek answers for myself. I began to do my own research and then I found some amazing things. The interesting thing is that I started to believe, I started to believe that maybe, just maybe we could help ourselves, heal ourselves and get a second chance to good health. What I find most difficult in this new love for health and wellness, however, is to convince others that there is hope for healing. Like the old saying goes, "You can lead a horse to water, but you can't make him drink."

Today I ask that as you read this guide, you would be open minded to new things, natural ideas and a renewed sense of hope for your own health. The body is so complex so it takes a lot of determination to feel better physically, especially as we age. **The mind, body and soul are definitely all connected and sometimes health is a lifetime journey.**

Join me as we travel down this road to health. Look forward and forget what is behind. It's a new day, a new breathe and a new way of thinking. Today is the first day of the rest of our lives, so let's enjoy it, shall we!

I pray that in all respects, you may prosper and be in good health,

Just as your soul prospers.

Introduction

HEALTH AND WELLNESS

GUIDE

A TO Z

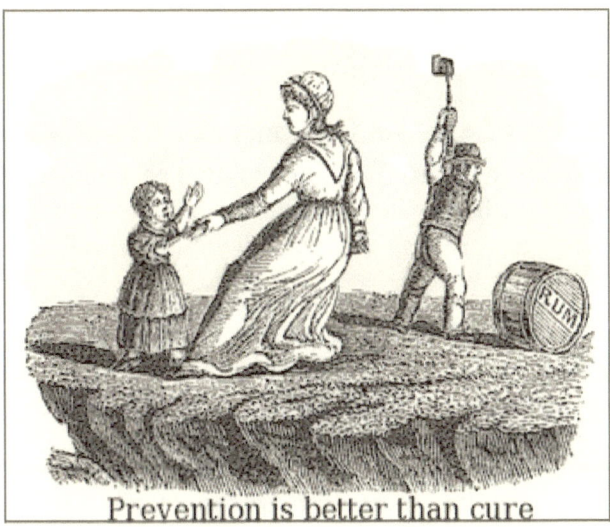

Prevention is better than cure

Prevention and wellness is better than cure. We must take care of ourselves **before** there is illness. How do we do this? This guide will give you practical steps to prevent disease as well as get back on the Health and Wellness road to recovery.

LET'S GET STARTED...

Step 1: **GO TO THE DOCTOR.** Do you know how many countless people procrastinate and put this off? I know that you are scared, but if you wait, your health could suffer. Have that blood, urine test and any others you might need. Just don't wait any longer! It could save your life.

Step 2: **START EATING HEALTHY EVERY DAY** Yes, I mean fruits and vegetables! You have heard it a million times, but real food, not packaged and processed food, brings life and healing. Everything you put into your mouth has a consequence—good or bad. Consider cutting out the soft drinks, especially the diet ones. Some research is suggesting there is a link with drinking them and depression, obesity, kidney damage, elevated blood pressure and stroke risk. Sugar should be avoided as much as possible as well.

"Let food be your medicine and medicine your food." Hippocrates

CONSIDER A PLANT BASED DIET *Forks over Knives*, a 2011 American documentary directed by filmmaker Lee Fulkerson, advocates a whole-food, plant-based diet as a means of combating a number of diseases including: coronary disease, diabetes, obesity, and cancer. It suggests that:

> ...**Most, if not all, of the degenerative diseases that afflict us can be controlled, or even reversed, by rejecting our present menu of animal-based and processed foods, including dairy.**
> **The China Study (1)**

IN THE *Forks over Knives* DOCUMENTARY,
THE RESEARCH FINDINGS WERE AMAZING.

One study looked at Norway during WWII when the Nazis came and occupied their country; they seized all cattle, pigs, and sheep from the Norwegians to feed the German army. During these years of occupation, the Norwegians were forced into a whole food, plant-based diet. **Heart disease and cancer in the Norwegians plummeted.** When the war was over and meat and dairy were re-introduced into their diets, these diseases returned.

A Is for Alternative Therapies

ELECTRO DERMAL SCREENING
AND
ZYTO COMPASS

How to assess health needs in addition to conventional means:

Electro Dermal Screening has its beginnings in what was called galvanic skin testing. The skin response is a method of measuring the electrical resistance of the skin and was discovered in the early 1900s. In the 1950s, a West German physician named Reinhold Voll combined acupuncture theory with galvanic skin response technology GSR. Galvanic skin testing detects sweat on the skin, and more sweat produces better electrical conduction. Voll tested the skin along various points with particular attention to the body's meridian as the patient holds a probe in one hand. The meridian energy flow carries with it information about internal organs that can be used in diagnosis. Through these skin-level measurements, it is possible to analyze the bio-energy and bio-information produced by internal organs and systems.

ZYTO Technology uses the same Galvanic Skin Response GSR technology to measure the fluctuations in electrical conductivity of the skin. In this method the client places their hand on a hand cradle and the software used sends stimuli to the body using digital signatures. Fluctuations in the Galvanic Skin Response are then measured and interpreted. The response helps to assess the health needs of the client. **Not for people with pacemakers. (2)

APPLE CIDER VINEGAR An apple a day can keep the doctor away because apples are full of healthy antioxidants, fiber, vitamins and minerals. One medium sized apple contains 4.4 g of dietary fiber. In addition, an apple is a good source of potassium, iron, phosphorus, manganese, calcium, magnesium and zinc. Apples also contain vitamins A, B1, B2, B6, C, E, K, foliate, and niacin.

Vinegar is an ancient folk remedy, believed to relieve just about any ailment you can think of. Some studies have hinted that apple cider vinegar could help with conditions such as diabetes (blood sugar), issues with the heart and obesity. Some other claims suggest that vinegar is also good for the digestive track and ailments of the gut, as well as arthritis, killing bacteria, high blood pressure, headaches, chronic fatigue, burns, gout, shingles, yeast, diabetes, sore throat, sinus infections, alcohol detox, endurance and even disinfectant use. (3)

Apple Cider Vinegar Drink:

- 1 ½ C. of filtered water
- 2 Tbsp. of juice and/or honey
- 2 Tbsp. of apple cider vinegar
- ½ tsp. of cinnamon

AMINO ACIDS are molecules that form protein. **Proteins are digested by the enzymes in the digestive tract turning them into amino acids.** Amino acids are fundamental nutrients that are indispensable to: components of protein, irreplaceable structural agents for muscles, chromosomes neurotransmitters, antibodies, sensory receptors and certain hormones. The body has a continual need for amino acids to create 2.5 million red blood cells every second to replace the blood platelets and the enterocytes (intestinal cells), and every 8 to 10 days to renew most of the leucocytes. The body needs these amino acids to: break down food, grow, and repair body tissue and many other bodily functions. To maximize the absorption of protein and amino acids we need to favor the antioxidants **and zinc** in our food or by supplementation. (4)

> **Collagen* If you lack the amino acids that combine to form collagen, your body's cells can't produce enough of it. Certain amino acids can be made in the body, but others must be provided by food. Thirty percent of our body is collagen and is a part of our tendons, ligaments, joints, muscles, hair, skin, and vital organs. Vitamin C is crucial to the creation of collagen. Creams are available for facials, and muscular, rheumatic and arthritic pains. Natural gelatin is also a great source of collagen.

12 essential amino acids are: Arginine, Histidine, Isoleucine, Leucine, Lysine, Methionine, Phenyl-alanine, Taurine, Threonine, Tryptophan, Tyrosine, Valine

ANTIOXIDANTS are substances that may protect your cells against the effects of **free radicals**. Free radicals are organic molecules responsible for damaging cells for aging, tissue damage, and some diseases. These molecules are very unstable and look to bond with other molecules, destroying their health and further continuing the damaging process. Antioxidants, present in many foods are molecules that prevent free radicals from harming healthy tissue. Free radicals are molecules produced when your body breaks down food, or by environmental exposures like tobacco smoke and radiation. Free radicals may play a role in heart disease, cancer and other diseases. Antioxidants are found in many foods: fruits, vegetables, nuts, grains, some meats, fish & poultry. **Alpha-Lipoic Acid ALA** is an impressive antioxidant. **Other antioxidants are:** Beta-carotene, Lutein, Lycopene, Selenium, Vitamin A, Vitamin C, and Vitamin E. Highest antioxidant values: cinnamon, clove, turmeric, red beans, blueberries, kidney beans.

THERE ARE CERTAIN WAYS WE CAN MEASURE HEALTH, HERE ARE THREE:

BLOOD PRESSURE

Blood Pressure	Optimal	Normal	High Normal	Hypertension
Systolic	Less than 120	Less than 130	130-139	140 or higher
Diastolic	Less than 80	Less than 85	85-89	90 or higher

BLOOD SUGAR

BLOOD GLUCOSE CHART			
Mg/DL	Fasting	After Eating	2-3 hours After Eating
Normal	80-100	170-200	120-140
Impaired Glucose	101-125	190-230	140-160
Diabetic	126+	220-300	200 plus

BODY MASS INDEX (BMI)

BMI uses your height and weight values to determine whether you are at risk for weight-related health problems. The lower your BMI, the lower your risk for health problems.

$$BMI = \frac{Weight\ in\ pounds \times 703}{Height\ in\ inches \times Height\ in\ inches}$$

Healthier Living Naturally

A body mass index (BMI) of 18.5 to 24.9 is considered healthy. A person with a BMI of 25 to 29.9 is considered overweight, and a person with a BMI of 30 or more is considered obese.

BRAIN HEALTH

"You are only as young as your oldest part."
Dr. Eric Braverman, MD

Dr. Eric Braverman believes identifying your body's aging parts is the key to slowing the aging process and getting back on the road to good health. As we age, he says that deficiencies in our hormones, vitamins and neurotransmitters such as Dopamine and Serotonin can affect our brain and body functions negatively.

"These deficiencies lead to weight gain, loss of energy, decrease in sexual function, fatigue, osteoporosis, sleep loss, memory loss and a host of other symptoms that are signs of aging and can lead to serious illness. Prevention and early intervention can help reduce the risk of illness and improve health. Minor and moderate deficits can be treated without medications and usually respond to a combination of natural, nutritional, hormonal and lifestyle changes."

Braverman believes that your brain chemical activity determines which foods you are compelled to eat, the speed of your metabolism, and your ability to stop eating and recognize when you are full. <u>Restoring or enhancing your dopamine, acetylcholine, GABA, or serotonin, or any combination of them, he says is the only way you will be able to lose weight effectively and keep it off permanently</u>.

Dr. Braverman has designed the *Age Print Quiz* and the *Brain Quiz* to help you discover where your body is deficient. You can take the tests, and the number of true answers will personally show

your deficiencies. He also gives his professional recommenda-
tions at www.pathmed.com.

- ❖ **Age Print Quiz:** Heart, Immune System, Thyroid, Metabolism, Bones, Menopause, Andropause (Men), Gastric.
  http://www.pathmed.com/pdf/age_print_quiz.pdf

- ❖ **Brain Quiz:** GABA, Acetylcholine, Serotonin, Dopamine
  http://pathmed.com/pdf/brain_quiz.pdf

BREATHING PROPERLY

**According to www.NormalBreathing.com, "Over 90% of
modern people suffer from breathing problems. The common
problems include chest breathing, mouth breathing, and hyperventilation, all of which reduce oxygen levels in body cells
and promote chronic diseases."**

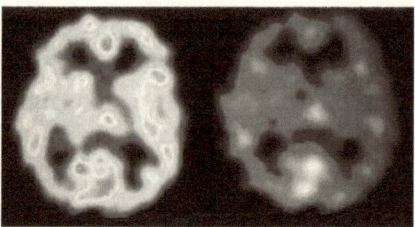

Photo: Normal Breathing versus Hyperventilation in the brain (5)

"Abnormally heavy breathing is possible to notice, and it causes
and promotes chronic diseases ranging from cancer and diabetes
to heart disease and obesity. In addition, chronic over breathing
creates problems with sleep, digestion, ability to exercise and
physical health. People with low body O2 generate free radicals,
have over-excited brains due to deficiency of all three brain chemicals: O2, CO2 and glucose. Therefore, they will suffer from panic

attacks, anxiety, addictions, inconsistent behavior, and other problems.

The **Buteyko Breathing** is a system of activities that include breathing exercises and lifestyle changes. The goal of the technique is to normalize or slow down one's *automatic or unconscious* breathing pattern or learn how to breathe in accordance with medical norms 24/7 so as to increase body and brain oxygenation."(5)

EMPTY NOSE SYNDROME
Have you ever had nasal surgery?

Do you struggle with breathing now? According to **www.emptynosesyndrome.org**, Empty Nose Syndrome (ENS), also known in research as "the wide nasal cavity syndrome," is a medical term used to describe a nose crippled by over resection of the inferior and/or middle turbinates of the nose resulting from surgery. The main symptoms are: chronic dryness of the nose and pharynx, shortness of breath, upsetting nasal sensations switching between over openness or congestion of the remaining mucosa, difficulty sleeping, difficulty concentrating and a generally depressed and irritated mood.

Did you know? According to D.C. Jarvis M. D. in his book, *Folk Medicine*, he says that chewing the honeycomb from honey is "excellent for treating certain disturbances of the **breathing tract as well inflammation of the sinuses**." Also, **chlorophyll or wheat grass** consumption increases the number of red blood cells and increases oxygen utilization by the body which could possibly help with breathing. Lastly, others have mentioned: hydrogen peroxide, coconut oil, N-acetylcysteine, bromelain, marshmallow root, mullein, wild cherry bark, horehound and ivy extract for lung, bronchial and sinus support. (See disclaimer)

CHIROPRACTIC CARE

Chiropractic care is an alternative medical system.

Your body has a powerful self-healing ability and the body's structure, mainly the spine and its function are related. The goal of chiropractic therapy is to normalize this relationship. Chiropractors or D. C. use hands-on therapy called spinal manipulation or an adjustment.

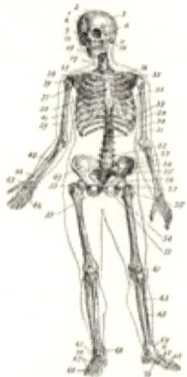

If you find a chiropractor that you are comfortable with and who listens to you, chiropractic adjustments or realignments can relieve pain and pressure throughout your body, especially your back and neck. We have nerves that surround the vertebrae and these nerves lead to vital organs, cells and glands that make the entire body, structure and immune system operate properly on a daily basis. When the immune system suffers interference, we can experience pain. Chiropractors usually emphasize management of the neuro-musculoskeletal system without the use of medicines or surgery.

"Healthy citizens are the greatest asset any country can have."
— Winston S. Churchill

DETOXIFY... WHY?

"Every day, our body is bombarded with harsh TOXINS and chemicals from our surrounding environment. Chemicals, pesticides, hormones and other pollutants are found in all the processed foods we eat, and often in the water we drink and the air we breathe. Although our bodies do have some built in means of expelling toxins, there are now so many different substances passing into our bodies that the toxic burden is proving too great for many to deal with properly. These harmful substances have accumulated to such an extent in many of us that chronic illnesses are proliferating at both the physical and mental levels. Under natural circumstances, the body is able to eliminate many of these toxic substances safely provided that is getting proper nutrition in sufficient quantities and the organs of detoxification are functioning at optimal levels. The main organs of detoxification are the skin, bowels, liver, kidney and lungs. In a natural habitat the human body will eliminate environmental toxins through perspiration, urination and bowel elimination." (6)

Not all detox programs require fasting. Some are very simple to do. It's natural and doesn't have to interfere with daily life either. Our bodies are around 70% water. Water is essential to detoxing. Drink 8-10 glasses of water daily to rid your body of the toxins. Be aware of any detoxing effects such as headaches and bowel changes.

Parasites

Did you know? According to the Center for Disease Control and Prevention there are *five* parasitic infections that have been neglected to be recognized in the United States. These infections cause serious illnesses, including seizures, blindness, infertility, heart failure, and even death. Millions of people in the U. S. could be affected and not know it.

Parasitic infections are typically associated with poor and often marginalized communities in low-income countries.

Healthier Living Naturally

However, these infections are also present in the United States. These infections are considered neglected because relatively little attention has been devoted to their surveillance, prevention, and/or treatment. Anyone, regardless of race or economic status, can become infected. (7)

Neglected Parasitic Infections include:

- **Chagas Disease** is transmitted to animals and people by insect vectors
- **Cysticercosis** is a parasitic tissue infection caused by larval cysts of the pork tapeworm
- **Toxocariasis** is the parasitic disease caused by the larvae of two species of Toxocara roundworms
- **Toxoplasmosis** is considered to be a leading cause of death attributed to foodborne illness in the United States.
- **Trichomoniasis** is a common sexually transmitted disease (STD) that is easy to cure.

Side effects of Parasitic Infections: migraines, insomnia, joint pain, fatigue, muscle pain, irritable bowel, disease, etc.

Possible Remedies: anti-fungal homeopathics, detoxing, Pau D'arco, proteolytic enzymes, sea salt cleanses, silver sol.

Fungus causes a wide variety of diseases in humans. Many fungi are good and useful (edible mushrooms would be an example) while some cause problems in people's health. Possible remedies: coconut oil, oregano oil, silver sol.

"Their fruit will be for food and their leaves for medicine."
Ezekiel 47:12

DIET

There are so many different diets to choose from, but this book is really about lifestyle change. You can find a diet that fits your health needs best, but the bottom line is that changing your diet to eat 100% healthy is something that you must buy into. The "light has to go on" that this is no longer an option, but a way of life that is necessary to improve the quality of your life.

Remember to eat three balanced meals a day-preferably eating the biggest meal before 3 p.m., chew your food well, eat reasonable portions, and actually sit down and take your time to eat. Don't eat three hours before bedtime if possible.

What is a healthy diet? Here are some ideas: Lots of fruits, vegetables, whole grains, brown rice, whole wheat pasta, rice cakes, popcorn, seeds, nuts, legumes such as kidney, pinto, black, white beans, split beans, lentils and black-eyed peas and nut butters, oils such as olive oil, coconut oil and spices.

Did you know?
- There are 4 calories in 1 gram of carbohydrates.
- There are 4 calories in 1 gram of protein.
- There are 9 calories in 1 gram of fat.
- There are 7 calories in 1 gram of alcohol.

If you ate a meal where the first food item (i.e. noodles) was 200 carbs that would equal to 800 calories; 50 g. of protein (i.e. meat) would equal to 200 calories, and 167 g. of fat would equal 1,503 calories. Your main dish alone would total 2503 calories!

"The doctor of the future will give no medicine, but will interest his patients in the care of the human frame, in diet and in the cause and prevention of disease."
Thomas Edison

ENVIRONMENTAL FRIENDLY PRODUCTS

We use or take in chemicals every day, whether it's in cleaning, gardening, applying cosmetics, body and hair products or just breathing. These chemicals are known to change our physical health and over time the human body accumulates these toxins. These bacteria and germs, if left unchecked, can add up. The best way to take care of these harmful chemicals stored in the body is through detoxification, and maybe we need to make some life-style changes as well. Many natural products can do the same job or better than the man-made versions. For example, vinegar, baking soda and hydrogen peroxide are great cleaning agents. Natural cosmetics are often from fruit which are antioxidants. Natural hair and body products can also be purchased for the same cost usually as regular brands. *Consider natural products to support your body's health.*

ENZYMES

The term enzyme comes from the Greek word,
Zymosis, which means fermentation.

Enzymes are catalysts which help in the digestion and assimilation of nutrients. They are crucial for building up the immune response.

There are 3 kinds of enzymes:
1. *Metabolic* are primarily in charge of energy production in the body. They also help to detox the body on a cellular level and help the sensory system respond appropriately. They are responsible for cellular activity on every level and help with metabolism.

2. *Digestive* who assist the body with breaking down and assimilating food into nutrients. The body uses different types of enzymes to digest fats, proteins and carbohydrates. (*You can buy enzymes in pill form to aid with digestion.*)

3. *Food Enzymes* that primarily come from plants. Our body cannot make these enzymes, but are contained in the food we eat. Our body breaks down the food, but enzymes are destroyed by heat so it is important to eat fresh raw fruit and vegetables and not just cooked ones.

Our body cannot function without enzymes. We have a limited supply and our bodies cannot produce all the enzymes we need. They are destroyed by: stress, poor diet, heat, microwaving, meat tenderizing, sterilization, pasteurization, antibiotics, chemotherapy, pesticides, preservatives, ibuprofen, pH and aspirin. Since the tight control of enzyme activity is essential for homeostasis or a stable state, any malfunction (mutation, overproduction, underproduction or deletion) of a single critical enzyme can lead to a genetic disease. Zinc helps in the activation of enzymes. (Zinc sources: oysters, shellfish, red meats, whole grains.) Magnesium is also essential for enzyme production. **The importance of enzymes is shown by the fact that a lethal illness can be caused by the malfunction of just one type of enzyme out of the thousands of types present in our bodies.** Oral administration of enzymes can be used to treat several diseases (e.g. pancreatic insufficiency, lactose intolerance, etc.) (8)

Good sources of enzymes:
✓ Fresh fruit and vegetables
✓ Seeds, nuts, grains and beans
✓ Fermented foods: kefir, sauerkraut, soy sauce, yogurt, pickles.

Prevention is better than cure. -Desiderius Erasmus

ESSENTIAL NUTRIENTS

Essential nutrients are vital for every bodily function, from building healthy bones and teeth, to energy production, to immune support. Minerals are so crucial to our health that even a slight imbalance of one mineral can have major consequences. It is important that the essential nutrients put into one's body are **plant-derived** phyto-nutrients, pure, synthetic-free, pesticide-free, and does not contain any preservatives, inorganic compounds, or animal products. Additives such as yeast, corn, wheat, soy, or dairy should be avoided as well.

HERE ARE 91 ESSENTIAL NUTRIENTS THAT WE NEED:

60 Essential Minerals (organic not synthetic)

Aluminum, Arsenic, Barium, Beryllium, Boron, Bromine, Carbon, Calcium, Cerium, Cesium Chloride, Chromium Cobalt, Copper, Dysprosium, Erbium, Europium, Gadolinium, Gallium, Germanium, Gold, Hafnium, Holmium, Hydrogen, Iodine, Iron, Lanthanum, Lithium, Lutetium, Magnesium, Manganese, Molybdenum, Neodymium, Nickel, Niobium, Nitrogen, Oxygen, Phosphorus, Potassium, Praseodymium, Rhenium, Rubidium, Samarium, Scandium, Selenium, Silica, Silver, Sodium, Strontium, Sulfur, Tantalum, Terbium, Thulium, Tin, Titanium, Vanadium, Ytterbium, Yttrium, Zinc, Zirconium.

16 Essential Vitamins:

Vitamin A, Vitamin B1 (Thiamine), Vitamin B2 (Riboflavin), Vitamin B3 (Niacin), Vitamin B5 (Pantothenic Acid), Vitamin B6 (Pyridoxine), Vitamin B12 (Cobalamin), Vitamin C, Vitamin D, Vitamin E, Vitamin K, Biotin, Choline, Flavonoids and Bioflavonoids, Folic Acid, Inositol.

12 Essential Amino Acids

Arginine, Histidine, Isoleucine, Leucine, Lysine, Methionine, Phenylalanine, Taurine, Threonine, Tryptophan, Tyrosine, Valine

3 Essential Fatty Acids

Omega 3, Omega 6, Omega 9

ESSENTIAL OILS

Essential oils have been used medicinally all throughout history and have been used to heal physical ailments. Essential oils are **concentrated** liquid compounds distilled from plants. Some oils can be ingested, used for massage, or diffused as incense; they are also put into soaps, perfumes and even cleaning products. Typically, essential oils are diluted with a carrier oil such as rose oil.

Pure, therapeutic grade is the best. There are too many oils to list here, but these are worth mentioning. They should be used with proper instruction and tested first for allergies. *Not all purposes are listed or proven by science.*

- ❖ **Bergamot** acne, psoriasis, stress, urinary & digestive health
- ❖ **Black Pepper** digestion, intestinal health, endurance, energy
- ❖ **Cinnamon** diabetes, obesity, arthritis, high cholesterol, blood pressure, urinary tract, stomach issues
- ❖ **Clove** asthma, chest infections, respiratory, warts, cuts, bruises
- ❖ **Eucalyptus** antibacterial, arthritis, respiratory, muscle pain, migraine

- ❖ **Geranium** circulatory system, cold sores, PMS, menopause, skin problems
- ❖ **Ginger** allergies, arthritis, circulatory, backache, cold & flu, lymphatic, motion sickness
- ❖ **Grapefruit** acne, muscle fatigue, antiseptic, detoxification, menstrual
- ❖ **Helichrysium** bruising, varicose veins, circulatory health & muscle tension
- ❖ **Lavender** skin issues, burns, relaxation, mood swings, insect repellant, sunburn, allergies
- ❖ **Lemon** anemia, digestion, kidney, colds, removing pesticides from fruits and vegetables
- ❖ **Oregano "medicine cabinet all in one"** antibiotic, and good for a ton of other things.
- ❖ **Tea Tree (Melaleuca)** asthma, athlete's foot, chicken pox blemishes, cold sores, skin issues, warts
- ❖ **Peppermint** heart palpitations, migraines memory, digestion, fatigue, arthritis, cramps, and colds
- ❖ **Rose** allergies, anger, anxiety, circulation, depression, menstruation, asthma
- ❖ **Ylang Ylang** anxiety, rapid heartbeat & breathing, mild food poisoning, intestinal health

BIBLICAL OILS: Calamus, Cassia (Cinnamon), Cedarwood, Cypress, Frankincense (Boswellia)*, Galbanum, Hyssop, Myrrh, Myrtle, Onycha, Rose of Sharon, Sandalwood, Spikenard.

EXERCISE

We have all heard how beneficial exercise can be. Make an effort today to get out and get on your feet. Grab a friend to exercise with you if you can, this makes exercise a little more fun. And each time you do exercise, try to do it a little longer. Ideally, you should exercise at least three times weekly for a minimum of 20

Healthier Living Naturally

minutes a day, incorporating *aerobic, range of motion and resistance* into it. Don't beat yourself up if you miss a day or two. You'll do better next week, just DON'T give up!

Exercise can be defined within three categories according to the American College of Sports Medicine:

1. **Aerobic** - cardiovascular exercise, such as running on a treadmill or cycling.

2. **Range of Motion** – this is basically stretching each muscle group for 30 seconds to increase range of motion for ligaments, tendons and muscles.

3. **Resistance** – this has to do with weights or machines with the expectation of increasing one's strength, tone, mass, and endurance.

[HEART RATE]

How to determine your MAXIMUM HEART RATE (MHR) in exercise:

❖ 220 – your age = Your MAXIMUM HEART RATE

How to determine your MINUMUM HEART RATE in exercise:

❖ Your MAXIMUM HEART RATE x .50 = Your Minimum Heart Rate

How to determine you 10-second target heart rate:

❖ Divide your Minimum Heart Rate by 6

Resting Heart Rate for WOMEN						
Age	18-25	26-35	36-45	46-55	56-65	65+
Athlete	54-60	54-59	54-59	54-60	54-59	54-59
Excellent	61-65	60-64	60-64	61-65	60-64	60-64
Good	66-69	65-68	65-69	66-69	65-68	65-68
Above Average	70-73	69-72	70-73	70-73	69-73	69-72
Average	74-78	73-76	74-78	74-77	74-77	73-76
Below Average	79-84	77-82	79-84	78-83	78-83	77-84
Poor	85+	83+	85+	84+	84+	84+

Resting Heart Rate for MEN						
Age	18-25	26-35	36-45	46-55	56-65	65+
Athlete	49-55	49-54	50-56	50-57	51-56	50-55
Excellent	56-61	55-61	57-62	58-63	57-61	56-61
Good	62-65	62-65	63-66	64-67	62-67	62-65
Above Average	66-69	66-70	67-70	68-71	68-71	66-69
Average	70-73	71-74	71-75	72-76	72-75	70-73
Below Average	74-81	75-81	76-82	77-83	76-81	74-79
Poor	82+	82+	83+	84+	82+	80+

Remember... EXERCISE controls weight, combats disease, improves mood and energy, promotes better sleep and connects you socially with people.

FATTY ACIDS These essential fatty acids Omega-3, 6 and 7 are *good* for you. Without them, you could cause serious damage to different systems within your body. They are not usually produced naturally within our body and you have to get them by adding them to your diet. **Omega-3 sources:** salmon, tuna, trout, sardines, coconut and canola oil, walnuts & flaxseed. **Omega-6 sources:** vegetable oils, nuts, whole wheat bread and chicken.

Omega-7 has numerous skin and health benefits, but it is also known for its ability to support a healthy weight, cardiovascular health, and gastro-intestinal health. **Omega-7** can be found in animal and plant sources, including: macadamia nuts, cold-water fish and sea buckthorn berries. Be careful to balance your intake of these fatty acids.

FIBER OR PSYLLIUM a 2011 study reported by the National Institutes of Health found that those who consumed higher amounts of fiber over a nine-year period had a significantly less chance of dying from chronic disease than those who consumed less fiber. Fiber consumption of study participants ranged from 12.6 g to 29.4 g per day in men and from 10.8 to 25.8 g per day in women. **Those who consumed the most fiber each day had a 22 percent lower risk of death over the nine-year period than those who consumed the least amount of fiber.** Fiber can be found in fruits and vegetables and will improve bowel function and lower bad cholesterol.

FRUIT...GOOD FOR YOU!

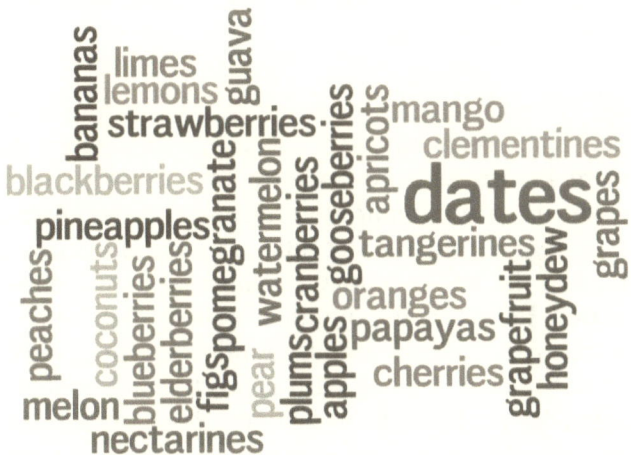

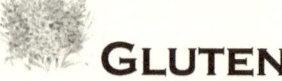

GLUTEN

Reports indicate gluten intolerance has quadrupled in the last 50 years.

Gluten is a protein composite found in foods processed from wheat and related grain species, including barley and rye. Celiac disease is an abnormal immune reaction to partially digested gliadin. There are also wheat allergies. Gluten can be found in pasta, cold cuts, salad dressings, beer, and even licorice. It can cause a number of ailments such as: gas, bloating, acid reflux, fatigue, irritable bowel, diarrhea, chronic constipation, headaches, joint pain, brain fog, anemia, osteoporosis, and in extreme cases, lymphoma. If you have these symptoms after eating, making a dietary change could be essential. Some grains and starches allowed in a gluten-free diet include: corn, quinoa, rice, tapioca, buckwheat. Also allowed are fresh meats, fish and poultry, fruits, potatoes, vegetables, wine and cider. Peppermint oil can help relieve esophageal spasms. [See information on **Probiotic: Bifidobacteria and GMOs.**]

On February 24, 2013, The New York Times reported some interesting research on gluten:

> Dr. Yolanda Sanz, a researcher at the Institute of Agrochemistry and Food Technology in Valencia, Spain noted that the bacterium known as bifidobacteria was depleted in children with celiac disease, compared to healthy children. Also present were strains of E. coli. In a test tube, Dr. Sanz found that the E. coli enhanced the inflammatory response of human intestinal cells to gluten. However, the bifidobacteria changed the response from inflammation to tolerance. Bifidobacteria occurs naturally in breast milk, and along with protective antibodies and immune-signaling proteins, brings hundreds of prebiotic sugars. These sugars selectively feed certain microbes in the infant gut, but particularly bifidobacteria. Bifidobacteria exist more in breast-fed infants than formula-fed ones.

In an effort to prevent celiac disease, parents were instructed to delay the introduction of gluten until their babies were six months old. That also happened to be when many Swedish mothers weaned their children. Coincidentally, companies had increased the amount of gluten in baby food. "Dr. Sanz noted that a group of bacteria native to the intestine known as bifidobacteria were relatively depleted in children with celiac disease compared with healthy controls. Other microbes, including native E. coli strains, were overly abundant and oddly virulent."

Dr. Anneli Ivarsson, a pediatrician at Umea University, found that the longer children breast-fed after their first exposure to gluten, the more protected they were... But it's a secondary observation that has Dr. Alessio Fasano, head of the Center for Celiac Research and Treatment at the Massachusetts General Hospital for Children in Boston, particularly intrigued. He said, "Two of these children developed autoimmune disease: one celiac disease, another, Type 1 diabetes, which shares genetic susceptibility with celiac disease. In both cases, a decline of lactobacilli preceded disease onset." (9)

HAIR ANALYSIS OR SALIVA TESTING

These tests can measure the levels of trace minerals in the body. Trace minerals are essential for our internal metabolic function and provide the building blocks to life, but are also necessary in hormone and enzyme activity. The body can manufacture many vitamins, but it cannot produce essential trace minerals. We rely on food to give us these. Because our soils are depleted of vital minerals, our foods are starved of nutrition as well. Many health symptoms are part of mineral deficiencies, imbalances or toxic accumulation. The individual information gained through hair tissue mineral analysis can become an important tool to maintaining good health. **Sea Salt is a good source of trace minerals.**

HORMONE BALANCE

It is strongly recommended that you be evaluated by your physician before self-prescribing for hormone-related problems.

Hormonal balance is essential to healthy living. There is so much to understand about balancing hormones that it is difficult to know where to begin. Smart health may be to have your hormone levels tested periodically, just like a mammogram or Pap smear. But imbalances have serious consequences and if not kept in check, chances of cancer increase. Many cancers are hormone related. Estrogen dominance may be accountable for breast, prostate, cervix, endometrial, uterine, and ovarian cancer.

Many researchers attribute the high incidence of cancers to the presence of environmental estrogens in our food and products today. *Phytoestrogens* are plant-derived *xenoestrogens* and are consumed by eating phytoestrogenic plants. They *imitate estrogen, but are* not generated within the endocrine system; Phytoestrogens can be either synthetic or natural chemical compounds.

**Bioidentical Hormone
Replacement Therapy (BHRT)**
Also known as a natural alternative hormone therapy refers to the use of hormones that are identical, on a molecular level, with endogenous hormones in hormone replacement therapy.

Xenoestrogens: artificial scents, air fresheners, food additives, preservatives, commercially raised poultry and cattle, household cleaners, detergents, car exhaust and indoor toxins, personal care products (shampoos, lotions, perfumes, make up, deodorants), oral contraceptives, prescription drugs, paints, lacquers and solvents, pesticides, herbicides, fertilizers, Styrofoam products, plant estrogens (soy, flaxseed), **plastics,** canned foods, and plastic food wrap.

Healthier Living Naturally

Naturally Estrogenic: alcohol, alfalfa, anise seed, apples, barley, beets, black-eyed peas, blue/black cohosh, cherries, chickpeas, clover, cucumbers, dairy, dates, dong quai, eggs, eggplant, fennel, flaxseed, flour, garlic, hops, lavender, licorice, meat, oats, olive oil, olives, papaya, parsley, peas, peppers, plums, pomegranates, poppy seed, potatoes, pumpkin, red beans, red clover, rhodiola, rose root, rhubarb, rice, sage, saw palmetto, sesame seeds, soybean, sprouts, sugar, sunflower seeds, tea tree oil, tomatoes, wheat, white rice., soy, canola, safflower and corn oil.

Foods That Inhibit Estrogen: artichoke, asparagus, avocados, berries, brazil nuts, broccoli, buckwheat, cabbage, celery, citrus fruits (except apples, cherries, dates, pomegranates), figs, garlic, grapes, green beans, green tea, melons, nuts, onions, pears, pineapples, seaweed, squash, tapioca, white flour, white rice.

Balancing Hormones: carrots, chia seeds, coconut oil, cod liver oil, Diindolylmethane (DIM), false unicorn, gelatin, kelp, maca root, magnesium, olive leaf extract, parsley, quinoa, red raspberry, Vitamin D.

Increases Progesterone: beta carotene, chaste berry, dill, legumes, natural creams, oregano, seeds, sweet potato, thyme, turmeric, vegetables, Vitamin B6, C & E, L-arginine, wild yam.

Symptoms of Hormone Imbalance	
Women	**Men**
☐ Mood swings	☐ Burned out feeling
☐ Hot flashes	☐ Abdominal fat
☐ Night sweats	☐ Prostate problems
☐ Fatigue	☐ Decreased mental clarity
☐ Headaches	☐ Decreased sex drive
☐ Depressed	☐ Increased urinary urge
☐ Anxious	☐ Decreased strength
☐ Nervous	☐ Decreased stamina
☐ Irritable	☐ Difficulty sleeping
☐ Tearful	☐ Decreased urine flow
☐ Memory Lapse	☐ Irritable
☐ Weight gain	☐ Depression
☐ Premature aging	☐ Erectile dysfunction
☐ Vaginal dryness	☐ Hot flashes
☐ Heavy menses	☐ Night sweats
☐ Bleeding changes	☐ Poor concentration
☐ Incontinence	
☐ Fibrocystic breast	
☐ Decreased sex drive	
☐ Tender breast	
☐ Osteoporosis	
☐ Water retention	

http://youthfulagingcenter.com/estrogen-and-menopause.html

INFLAMMATION is often created by eating large quantities of sugar and bad fats. Inflammation affects brain chemistry and is one of the primary sources of aging, infections, autoimmune deficiencies and cancer. It is one of the hidden triggers to cardiovascular disease, increasing your risk for heart attack and stroke; it also affects metabolism and the skin.

Some other examples of inflammation would be: Arthritis, Bursitis, Carpal Tunnel, frostbite and Tendonitis. A product such as Penetrex™ delivers Arnica, Boswellia Serrata (Frankincense), Cetyl Myristoleate, Shea Butter, MSM (DMSO) and Vitamin B6 to the muscles, nerves, ligaments and tendons and can possibly counteract this inflammation. See your physician first.

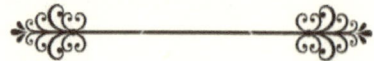

IODINE is necessary for the thyroid's gland performance. All blood of the body passes through the gland every 17 minutes and has a need for iodine. During the blood's passage, the gland's secretion of iodine kills weak germs that may have gained entry into the throat or through absorption of food from the digestive tract. Strong germs become weaker during the passage. If there is a normal supply of iodine, the germs are finally killed. If there is not, it cannot kill harmful germs circulating in the blood. A *second function* of iodine is to calm the body and relieve nervous tension. According to D. C. Jarvis' book, *Folk Medicine* p. 139, he was able to calm impatient and restless children under the age of 10 within two hours, giving them one drop of iodine by mouth in fruit juice. The *third function* according to Jarvis is that iodine can cause clear thinking. Deficiency is said to sometimes cause retardation, lower IQ, learning disabilities and miscarriage. **Cod liver oil** is rich in iodine as well as most food out of the ocean, radishes, asparagus, carrots, tomatoes, spinach, rhubarb, potatoes, peas, strawberries, mushrooms, lettuce, bananas, cabbage, egg yolk and onions.

Healthier Living Naturally

Juicing We should get at least 7 servings of fruits and vegetables per day, but very few of us actually do. Juicing or creating a favorite **smoothie** is an easy way to reach your daily target and helps you absorb the nutrients in a quick way. Add a wide variety of fruits and vegetables and start juicing with the ones you like first. Examples: celery, spinach, wheat grass, kale, collard greens, carrots and beets, lemon, limes, cranberries, bananas, apples, etc. Organic is best; wash with filtered water and lemon juice and leave the peels. Consider adding a protein powder with fruits and vegetables to add to the number of servings.

Kelp Hypothyroidism, which can bring about a slow metabolism and even weight gain, is often related to an iodine deficiency. *Kelp or seaweed* is a food that has been found effective in combating fat absorption, more so than some fat blockers sold in stores. Kelp could be something to consider when obesity is an issue. Other health problems that kelp could possibly help with are: heart and respiratory health, kidney function, indigestion, headaches, stress, depression, energy and ulcers. Seaweed is also highly alkaline so it can help improve pH levels. **Since cancer will only thrive in an acidic environment, seaweed is a great option to improve one's health.**

Ketone Ester-Containing Diet: Coconut Oil and Improved Cognitive Function

PRECLINICAL TRIAL: Ketone Esters

"The present findings show that long-term feeding of ketone esters not only improved behavioral cognitive function but also decreased Ab and pTau pathologic changes. The increase in blood ketone bodies, by either a ketogenic diet or by feeding a ketone ester, would be expected to alleviate the impaired brain glucose metabolism that precedes the onset of **Alzheimer's disease.** Our preclinical findings suggest that a ketone ester-containing diet has the potential to retard the disease process and improve cognitive function of patients with AD."

(Source:http://www.coconutketones.com/pdfs/Kashiwaya_Y_NeurobiolofAging_2012.pdf)

Healthier Living Naturally

According to Livestrong... Ketones are molecules that your heart, brain and muscles can use for energy, instead of sugar or fat. Most of your cells are actually 25 percent more efficient when using ketones instead of sugar. Ketones are not present in foods. Although ketones are a source of energy that almost all of your body cells can use, ketones are actually a byproduct of fat oxidation. In other words, when your body burns fat, it produces ketones that can be used for energy. The more your body burns fat, the more ketones produced.

The foods you choose can help you promote ketosis or the state in which your body uses ketones. To get your body to produce ketones, you need to follow a very low-carb, moderate protein and high fat diet. A Ketone Ester-Containing Diet might be: eggs cooked in generous amounts of olive oil, cheese, sausages, spinach, mushrooms and cherry tomatoes; fish, chicken or steak cooked in generous quantities of coconut oil, along with asparagus.

Coconut oil contains a type of fat called medium-chain triglycerides or MCTs that promote the production of ketones. Just as diabetics have problems with glucose and insulin, so Alzheimer's sufferers cannot get enough glucose into brain cells to give them the energy they need to lay down new memories and think clearly. *See your physician before starting any program.

Coconut Use Guidelines according to Dr. Mary T. Newport: Dr. Mary T. Newport, whose own husband's Alzheimer's condition improved by using coconut, says that coconut oil can be substituted for any solid or liquid oil, lard, butter or margarine in baking or cooking on the stove, and can be mixed directly into foods already prepared. She recommends 1 teaspoon with your meal and increasing slowly as tolerated. Coconut oil has about 117-120 calories per tablespoon, about the same as other oils. It contains 57-60% medium chain triglycerides (MCT), which are absorbed directly without the need for digestive enzymes.

Who should try this? People who have a neurodegenerative disease that involves decreased glucose uptake in neurons could benefit from taking higher amounts of coconut oil to produce ketones which may be used by brain cells as energy. These diseases include Alzheimer's and other dementias, Parkinson's, ALS (Lou Gehrig's), Multiple Sclerosis, Duchenne Muscular Dystrophy, Autism, Down's syndrome, and Huntington's chorea.

*For more information: http://coconutketones.com/; Clinical Trial: University of South Florida (USF) Byrd Alzheimer Institute 2013.

Leaky Gut Syndrome
All diseases start in the gut. Hippocrates

Symptoms: inflammation, bloating, gas, cramps, fatigue, joint pain, eczema

Causes of Leaky Gut Syndrom: food sensitivities, allergies, artificial sweetners, soft drinks, antibiotics, high sugar diet, parasites, stress, NSAIDS (ibuprofen, aspirin).

What is Leaky Gut Syndrome? This syndrome occurs when the digestive lining of the intestines becomes damaged and permeable. When this occurs, the bacteria, undigested food particles, toxic waste and viruses can leak from the intestines through the digestive lining *into the bloodstream*. In response, our immune system reacts negatively, which can result in inflammation in the body. Bloating, food sensitivities which appear like allergies, achy joints, cramps, headaches, rashes, and hives can appear. This condition may potentially create or worsen a number of other conditions, including: asthma, arthritis, Celiac disease, Crohn's, colitis, eczema, irritable bowel syndrome (IBS), inflammatory bowel disease and psoriasis. With leaky gut, not only is the digestive lining more porous and less selective about what can get in, but normal absorption is affected. Nutritional deficiencies may develop as a result of damage and the intestines are not able to absorb the vitamins and nutrients that the body needs.

Scientists are learning that **serotonin** made by the nervous system might also play a role in the gut. In a new *Nature Medicine* study published online February 7, 2010, it said, "a drug that inhibited the release of serotonin from the gut counteracted the bone-deteriorating disease osteoporosis in postmenopausal rodents... Serotonin seeping from the second brain (the gut) might even play some part in autism, the developmental disorder often first noticed in early childhood." Dr. M. Gershon has discovered that the same genes involved in synapse formation between neurons in the brain are involved in the alimentary synapse formation. "If these genes are affected in autism," he says, "it could explain why so many kids with **autism** have GI motor abnormalities" in addition to <u>elevated levels of gut-produced serotonin in their blood</u>." (10)

> **Gut and Psychology Syndrome GAPS** Dr. Campbell-McBride of Cambridge Nutrition Clinic in the UK, believes that abnormal gut flora can affect your brain and your entire body. Bacteria, yeast, viruses and other microbes that rage unchecked in the digestive tract can cause devastating consequences. Dr. Campbell-McBride believes autistic children are born with normal brains and normal sensory organs. She believes that during birth, and as a baby goes through the birth canal, he or she swallows the first mouthfuls of bacteria and that becomes the baby's gut flora, originating from antibiotics, birth control pills, and even the father's bacteria. No matter what symptoms an adult or child may experience, diet is the place to start according to Dr. Campbell-McBride. In 2004, she published *Gut and Psychology Syndrome: Natural Treatment of Autism, ADHD, Dyslexia, Dyspraxia, Depression and Schizophrenia*, in which she ex-

plores the connection between the patient's physical state and brain function.

Now What? First, get a Gastro Intestinal or GI test for verification purposes, then **BEGIN TO EAT RIGHT!** Consuming lots of anti-inflammatory essential fatty acids in fish and nuts, and filling up on green leafy vegetables, high-fiber and fermented foods help to promote the growth of good bacteria. A strong **probiotic*** with large amounts of good bacteria can heal a damaged intestinal lining by restoring balance in the gut flora. *Lactobacillus reuteri* and *Saccharomyces boulardii* is said to help children shorten the duration of infectious diarrhea, create a healthy flora and keep pathogens from passing through the intestinal wall to the rest of the body, as well as boost the immune system. For adults, consider *S. boulardii, Lactobacillus acidophilus* and *Bifidobacterium.* **(*See information on Probiotic: Bifidobacteria).**

Take Vitamin A or Cod Liver Oil to replenish deficiency of essential fatty acids. Supplements like glutamine, show that in some studies they help with intestinal injury after chemotherapy and radiation and may also be beneficial with leaky gut. Apple Cider Vinegar can help repair the gut, and taking digestive enzymes (pill form) can also be of benefit. By doing all these things, most people should notice improvement within 6 weeks, although it may take months or even years to heal a damaged intestinal lining in extreme cases of leaky gut.

MAGNESIUM It is estimated 80 % of Americans are deficient in this important mineral and the health consequences of deficiency are significant. Magnesium is the fourth most abundant mineral in the body and is essential to good health. Approximately 50% of total body magnesium is found in bone. The other half is found predominantly inside cells of body tissues and organs. Only 1% of magnesium is found in blood, but the body works very hard to keep blood levels of magnesium constant.

Healthier Living Naturally

Magnesium is needed for more than 300 biochemical reactions in the body. It helps maintain normal muscle and nerve function, keeps heart rhythm steady, supports a healthy immune system, and keeps bones strong. Magnesium also helps regulate blood sugar levels, promotes normal blood pressure, and is known to be involved in energy metabolism and protein synthesis. It is important in preventing and managing disorders such as hypertension, cardiovascular disease, and diabetes. Dietary magnesium is absorbed in the small intestines and excreted through the kidneys. It can be found in foods such as halibut, white beans, oat bran, spinach, cashews and Brazil nuts. (11)

MEDITATE FOR GOOD MENTAL HEALTH

Bodily disease, which we look upon as whole and entire within itself, may, after all, be but a symptom of some ailment in the spiritual part. —Nathaniel Hawthorne

There is a need to contemplate life, create visions and goals and connect spiritually. The dictionary defines meditate this way: to engage in thought; reflect, engage in devout religious contemplation, or quiescent spiritual introspection.

In a 2012 research study done by Harold G. Koenig at the Department of Medicine and Psychiatry at Duke University Medical Center entitled, *Religion, Spirituality, and Health: The Research and Clinical Implications* says the following:

> *Religious/spiritual beliefs and practices are commonly used by both medical and psychiatric patients to cope with illness and other stressful life changes. A large volume of research shows that people who are more R/S have better mental health and adapt more quickly to health problems compared to those who are less R/S. These possible benefits to mental health and well-being have physiological consequences that impact physical health, affect the risk of disease, and influence response to treatment.*

(Source: http://www.hindawi.com/journals/isrn.psychiatry/2012/278730/abs/)

MENTAL ILLNESS today is said to be our number one health concern in our country. Mental illness can be described or labeled by professionals in many ways including: depression, psychosis, OCD, PTS, GAD and many others. The root of a disease should always be pursued and that can be done by the work of a professional.

Here are a few questions to ponder as you evaluate your own mental wellbeing. **"Do you feel significant? Do you feel there is direction and purpose for your life? Do you feel loved?"** How many people today self-medicate their pain away through drugs and alcohol? Finding significance and love many times has a direct correlation to mental illnesses. Maybe the pain of the past also needs to be addressed for the sake of one's mental health.

Here are ten questions that we may ask ourselves if we are suffering mentally:

1. Am I fulfilled in life or at least moving forward towards a goal?
2. What mistakes or bad choices have I made in the past?
3. Can I correct these missteps or unproductive periods in my life and **transform my thoughts**?
4. Has my experiences in life made me a better person?
5. If not, what can I learn from these experiences?
6. Do I understand that I cannot always control life circumstances?
7. Do I believe that I do have control over my choices today and that I can contribute to society in some way and choose to be **thankful**?
8. Can I **forgive** myself, forgive others and forgive the past?
9. How do I define good mental health for me personally?
10. What can I do today to get help, take responsibility, move forward, and **give back** to society?

NEVER underestimate the POWER of the vegetable...

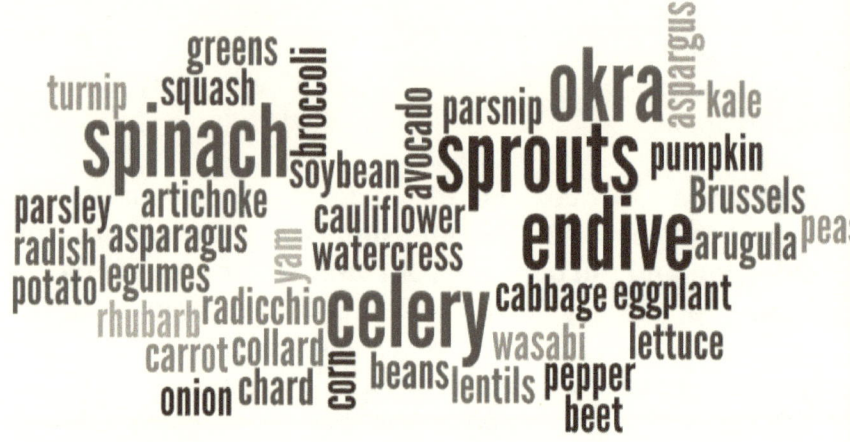

OTHER NOTABLE MENTIONS

❖ **Almond Milk** is usually soy and lactose free and is a milk alternative. 1 cup of milk can contain 276 mg. of calcium vs. 1 cup of Almond milk contains 467 mg. of calcium. **Coconut milk** is also a healthy option.

❖ **Aloe Vera Juice** is used for **pH balance** (gut), digestive issues, burns and eczema. It contains vitamins, minerals, sugars, enzymes, lignins, amino acids, anthraquinones, Saponins, essential fatty acids, salicylic acid, calcium, magnesium, zinc, vitamins A, B12 and E. It is considered an anti-inflammatory, anti-bacterial, and anti-viral. The inner gel of the *Aloe vera Barbadensis Miller plant* consists of more than 200 phytonutrients and the healing component, polymannans.

❖ **Bee Pollen, Royal Jelly, Propolis** - These are products supplied by bees and can be very effective in the fight against allergies, infertility, blood sugar and more.

❖ **Chanca Piedra** "stone breaker" can be used for kidney and gallstones; it can lead to an increase in urine output, and the excretion of sodium and creatine is enhanced. It is also known to have the ability to inhibit the creation of calcium oxalate crystals or stones.

- ❖ **Castor Oil** can be used for warts, moles, liver spots, newborn's navel, mother's breast to increase milk flow, eye irritation, longer eyelashes and eye brow growth, cuts, softens skin and calluses.
- ❖ **Cod Liver Oil** is an **omega-3 oil** and is considered "brain food" because it has been used to help treat conditions such as mental disorders or Alzheimer's disease. It has also been used for asthma and heart conditions.
- ❖ **Coconut Oil and Butter** helps with **dementia, Alzheimer's**, weight loss, skin, hair care, increased immunity and boosts energy level. Also strengthens bones and promotes a healthy digestive system and increases body's absorption of many beneficial substances such as calcium and magnesium. Coconut milk is a healthy milk substitute and is a medium chain fatty acid (easy to digest and burn as energy). *Unfortunately, because of the negative publicity of saturated fats, the benefits of coconut oil have been overlooked.
- ❖ **Echinacea** is antimicrobial; used for colds and flu, sore throats, immune system support, laxative, pain relief.
- ❖ **Fish Oil** is an **omega-3 oil** (good essential fatty acids) that is found in cold water fish, flaxseed, hemp and plant oils. They cannot be synthesized by the human body, but are vital for normal metabolism. Some evidence exists that it can be good for heart disease, varicose veins, blood pressure, inflammation, Alzheimer's & mental disorders.
- ❖ **Flaxseed oil** rich in **omega-3 fatty acids**, *alpha-linolenic acid*, is used to prevent and treat heart disease and to relieve a variety of inflammatory disorders (i.e. gout, lupus) and hormone-related problems-male and female, including infertility. Be aware of the phytoestrogens it contains. Not for pregnant women.
- ❖ **Gingko Biloba** is a leaf said to help with amyloidosis, memory (Alzheimer's), blood circulation, and heart health; prevents blood clotting and blood platelets from "sticking"

together. Protects the cells from free radicals and oxidative stress.

- ❖ **Honey** (dark) is a predigested sugar. **Bacteria cannot live in honey**. A copper source which unlocks many other vitamins and minerals, including Vitamin C. Good for: coughs (with lemon), hay fever, bedwetting, sleep, *cuts, burns,* cramps, twitching, digestion, fatigue, mosquito bites, endurance in sports. Not for children under one.

- ❖ **Hydrogen Peroxide "H2O2"** helps regulate the amount of oxygen getting to the cells. **Only 35% Food Grade hydrogen peroxide is recommended for internal use.** Helps a multitude of ailments, here are some: age spots, antiseptic, ear infections and wax, canker & cold sores, fungus, heart & lung issues, stamina, Epstein-Barr bacterial infections, liver cirrhosis, emphysema (Using vaporizer). *See disclaimer.*

- ❖ **Legumes** include: beans, peas, lentils, peanuts, and soybeans. Legumes are excellent sources of protein, low-glycemic index carbohydrates, essential micronutrients, and fiber.

- ❖ **Lemons** are antibacterial, antiviral, and immune-boosting and are a digestive aid and liver cleanser. The pH nature of lemons changes during the body's metabolic process and they become highly alkaline-forming. Adding just 1 tbsp. of fresh lemon juice to a glass of filtered water is an easy way to give your body a boost of alkalinity. Lemons are also great for the prevention of kidney stones.

- ❖ **Limes** health benefits include: weight loss, skin care, gout, gums, good digestion, eye care, relief from constipation, and treatment of scurvy, peptic ulcer, respiratory disorders, urinary disorders, piles, detoxes liver & gallbladder.

- ❖ **Maca** is a root native to the high Andes of Peru used for hormone balance, infertility (male/female), PMS, menopause, hot flashes, libido, energy, & anxiety.

- ❖ **Mustard** helps relaxes muscles, spasms, cramps (ingest); a decongestant (topically) and pain associated with burns; (seed) asthma, blood pressure, sleep.

❖ **Olive Oil** is a source of unsaturated fat or **omega-3** fatty acids which is good for your heart. Some experts believe that it can help prevent certain cancers and help lower blood sugar. Its antioxidant content is thought to help prevent digestive tract and prostate tumors.

> **Olive Leaf Extract** is known as a "Super food" and in many different studies has shown to be possibly effective with: athlete's foot, blood pressure regulation, cancer, cholesterol, heart health (arrhythmia and reduction in heart attack and stroke risk), chronic fatigue syndrome, fungi, molds, bladder infections, botulism, chicken pox, chlamydia, colds and flu, cold sores, diarrheal diseases, ear infections, E. coli, Epstein-Barr virus, fibromyalgia, food-borne illnesses, fungal infections, glucose homeostasis, hepatitis A, B and C, herpes, HIV virus, human papillomavirus (HPV), malaria, measles, meningitis, mumps, parasites, pelvic inflammatory disease, plague, pneumonia, polio, protozoans, rabies, ringworm, salmonella, sexually transmitted diseases, shingles, smallpox, streptococcus, tropical illnesses, tuberculosis, tumors, urinary tract infections, warts, and yeast infections.

❖ **Quinoa** (pronounced keen-wa) is an Omega 3 whole grain with zinc, vitamin E, and selenium that helps control weight and lower risk for heart disease and diabetes. **Groats** or **steel-cut oats** are the hulled grains of various cereals such as: oats, wheat, barley or rye. Groats are whole grains that include the cereal germ, the fiber-rich bran portion of the grain and the endosperm. *Both are gluten-free.*

❖ **Seeds & Nuts** are a great natural source of vitamins, minerals, protein, good fat, and fiber. Good for heart health as well. (i.e. chia, flax, *grape seed extract*, hemp, pumpkin, salba, sesame, sunflower; pistachios, almonds, walnuts and pecans).

❖ **Teas** have many health benefits; they have antioxidants and fight free radicals which are bad. Drinking 2-4 cups a day may offer curative and preventive health benefits from digestive issues to lowering blood pressure to helping fight against infections and boosting your metabolism. Four varieties are: green, black, white, and oolong. Anything else, like herbal tea is an infusion of different plants. *Flor Essence* is a tea whose properties fight cancer and other diseases.

❖ **Wheat Grass** is a food prepared from the cotyledons of the common wheat plant and provides **chlorophyll** (which increases the oxygen carrying capacity of the blood), amino acids, minerals, vitamins, and enzymes to the body. It is often served in juice bars alone, or in mixed fruit and vegetable drinks. **It contains no wheat gluten.**

pH Balance
Acidosis v. Alkalosis

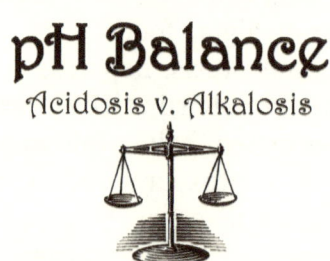

Does sickness come when the urine reaction is acid or alkaline?

Diseases thrive in an acidic, low oxygen environment. A mild alkaline pH solution has available over 100 times as much oxygen as a mild acidic solution. According to *Folk Medicine*, cancer could be an example of a disease that could grow in the wrong environment or acidosis. (12)

Most metabolic reactions in the body function within a balanced acid-alkaline pH range. Michael Romero, PhD of Mayo Clinic published research that states the body cannot function in either a state of acidosis or alkalosis. Foods and beverages affect the pH range of your body. Too much stress and lack of physical exercise can cause an increased acid pH in the body as well. Changing and adopting a healthier diet and lifestyle will help maintain an alkaline pH. According to D. C. Jarvis MD, author of *Folk Medicine*,

Healthier Living Naturally

"when there is a drop in the outdoor temperature, the blood reaction is also said to immediately become more alkaline, the adrenal gland is active, blood pressure rises and as the blood becomes more alkaline, tissue chemistry is altered. The reverse happens with warmer weather." **To maintain an alkaline environment in the body, experts suggest eating lots of fruits and vegetables which are sources of nutrients that can help maintain an alkaline environment...also eating fresh salads, seafood and fish.**

Body pH is measured on a scale of zero to 14, with 7.0 indicating neutral. Healthy pH ranges from 7.35 to 7.45, slightly alkaline, yet this level is conducive for maintaining metabolic processes. Excess acid in the blood, or acidosis, however, occurs when the pH falls below 7.35 and alkalosis occurs when pH is 7.45 or higher. A fruit and vegetable diet will move the pH balance to a more alkaline level by decreasing the amount of calcium eliminated from the body. To make your own alkaline water, simply squeeze lemon or lime into your filtered drinking water.

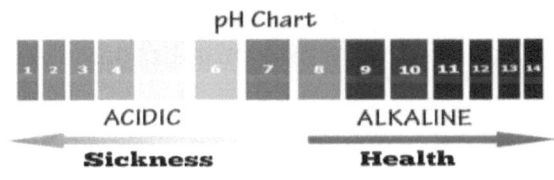

Testing: See your physician to determine initial pH levels with accuracy. Nitrazine paper is a pH indicator dye and is also available for purchase. Test your pH daily for two weeks, three times a day and record the results in a journal. Track the foods you eat. A urine pH test usually is the lowest in the morning. A pH near 7.3 indicates a healthy balance. Note that stress and anxiety, which can result in hyperventilation, can significantly increase the amount of carbon dioxide expelled into your bloodstream as well. A high level of carbon dioxide leads to alkalosis.

Potassium IS A VERY IMPORTANT MINERAL
TO THE HUMAN BODY.

According to National Institute for Health, your body needs potassium to: **build proteins, break down and use carbohydrates, build muscle, maintain normal body growth, control the electrical activity of the heart, help with brain function and control the acid-base balance.** (13)

Having too much or too little potassium in the body can have very serious consequences. **A low blood level of potassium is called hypokalemia.** It can cause weak muscles, abnormal heart rhythms, and a slight rise in blood pressure. You may have hypokalemia if you:

- Take diuretics (water pills) for the treatment of high blood pressure or heart failure
- Take too many laxatives
- Have severe or prolonged vomiting and diarrhea
- Have certain kidney or adrenal gland disorders
- **Foods good in potassium: white beans, spinach, baked potatoes, dried apricots, baked acorn squash, yogurt, salmon, avocados, white mushrooms, APPLE CIDER VINEGAR.**

Too much potassium in the blood is known as hyperkalemia. It may cause abnormal and dangerous heart rhythms. Some common causes include:

- Poor kidney function
- Heart medicines called angiotensin converting enzyme (ACE) inhibitors and angiotensin 2 receptor blockers (ARBs)
- Potassium-sparing diuretics (water pills) such as spironolactone or amiloride

PROBIOTIC: *Bifidobacteria*

Recent research shows "good bacteria" can actually lower blood pressure, prevent cancer, ease depression, and stop celiac. Prescription ANTIBIOTICS, however, kill good bacteria in our gut, as well as the second-hand consumption of antibiotics from beef, pork, dairy and poultry which contribute to poor flora in the G.I. Tract.

According to WebMd.com..."Bifidobacteria belong to a group of good bacteria called **lactic acid bacteria LAB** which are found in fermented foods. Bifidobacteria are used in treatment as "probiotics," the opposite of antibiotics. They are considered "friendly" bacteria. The human body counts on normal bacteria to break down foods, helping the body take in nutrients, and prevent the take-over of "bad" bacteria. Probiotics are typically used in cases when a disease occurs or might occur due to a kill-off of normal bacteria. Treatment with antibiotics can destroy disease-causing bacteria, but also normal bacteria in the gastrointestinal and urinary tracts." (14)

In a *2013 Health Radar* report it stated that probiotics may have a beneficial effect on the heart such as lowering cholesterol levels. **Further studies suggest that those with higher levels of good bacteria or probiotic microbes create anti-inflammatory compounds that keep plaque stable.** Remember, not all probiotics are created equally. Consider probiotics fermented over several years with seaweed, mushrooms, lactic acid, fruits, vegetables, vitamins, minerals, enzymes and amino acids and have at least 900 million CFUs.

Dr. Ohhira states that these probiotics help to keep us healthy by:

- ❖ Maintaining an appropriate digestive pH
- ❖ Supporting regularity
- ❖ Relieving the effects of occasional heartburn
- ❖ Making many of our vitamins
- ❖ Helping digest food

Healthier Living Naturally
- ❖ **Supporting the immune response**
- ❖ **Detoxing the body**
- ❖ **Balancing Hormones**

Did You Know? FDA warns that the antibiotics, **azithromycin "Z-pack" and levofloxacin (Levaquin) could lead to deadly heart rhythms for some patients.** According to the CBS news article, "The FDA is warning the public that the pills can cause abnormal changes in the heart's electrical activity that may lead to a fatal heart rhythm. Not everyone is at risk. Patients with known risk factors such as existing QT interval prolongation, low blood levels of potassium or magnesium, a slower than normal heart rate, or those who use certain drugs to treat abnormal heart rhythms, or arrhythmias face the greatest risk." The New England Journal of Medicine study was conducted at Vanderbilt University and re-vealed that patients who took the antibiotic were at a higher risk of developing heart problems. (15)

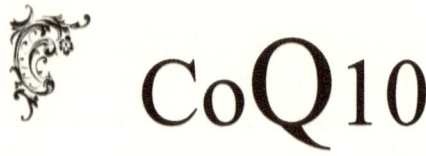

CoQ10

"The doctor of the future will give no medicine but will interest his patient in the human frame, in diet and the cause and prevention of disease." Thomas Edison

Coenzyme Q10 (CoQ10) is similar to a vitamin and is found in the cells of the body. Our bodies make CoQ10, and cells use it to produce body energy needed for cell growth and maintenance. It is an *antioxidant,* which protects the body from damage caused by harmful molecules and removes free radicals. CoQ10 is naturally present in small amounts in a variety of foods, but are particularly high in organ meats such as heart, liver, and kidney. Some other very important supplements for the heart include: **Crown of Thorns Extract (Hawthorn Berry)** which can be taken for

Healthier Living Naturally

chronic heart problems, **L-Arginine** which was the molecule of the year for heart in 1998 and creates Nitric Oxide and **Olive Leaf Extract** for arrhythmia. There is much research that indicates these supplements can help a multitude of heart ailments.

R & R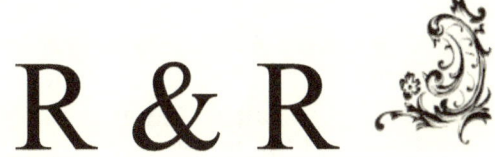

Early to bed and early to rise, makes a man healthy wealthy and wise.
Benjamin Franklin

Rest and relaxation is so much more important than we realize. Keeping stress levels down and getting better quality sleep makes us all healthier. (Try a little honey before bedtime). In the last forty years, the pace of our society has increased greatly. It used to be that on Sundays, it was a day of rest, going to church and visiting grandma. No more. Now there are tournament games that we HAVE to go to and worse yet, Sundays have been set aside to go to the grocery store and do laundry. Focus has been taken away from sitting at the kitchen table together to eating fast food in the car. No wonder why we are fatter and less healthy! But looking forward, we now need to make a lifestyle change...better rest, better food and better health. It's a decision. It won't look perfect, but it can be better. Take some time out for faith and family and then breathe slowly... and deeply. Take in the flowers and the sunshine and begin to count the blessings that you DO have...one blessing at a time.

In a disordered mind, as in a disordered body,
soundness of health is impossible. ~Cicero

Salt

Epsom, Dead Sea, Himalayan

It has been estimated that over 75% of the salt intake in the U.S. is derived from salt added during food processing or manufacturing, rather than from salt added at the table or during cooking. Sometimes "salt" and "sodium" is used interchangeably, but this is not correct. Table salt is sodium chloride and is 40% sodium and 60% chloride. Sodium is an essential nutrient; a mineral that the body cannot manufacture itself, but too much of anything, is not a good thing. Minerals and trace elements are found in salt. Iodized salt is preferred. Iodine deficiencies can cause cretinism, stillbirth, miscarriage, mental retardation and lower IQ.

- **Epsom salt or Magnesium sulfate is** an inorganic salt and originates from Surrey, England and is used internally and externally. The sulfate is also supplied in a gel preparation for topical application in treating aches and pains. Magnesium is used in multiple systems within the body. **According to some sources, it serves as a regulator for more than 325 enzymes in our bodies.** The sulfates in Epsom salt help the body absorb nutrients; flush out toxins and form proteins and muscle tissue. Also used in gardening as a soil supplement and in bath treatments. People, who are magnesium deficient, can have the following: heart disease, stroke, osteoporosis, arthritis and joint pain, digestive problems, and chronic fatigue. *Used to treat autism, inflammation, constipation, sprains, detox and more.*

- **Dead Sea** salts differ greatly from other sea salts in mineral content. Made up of only 8% sodium chloride with a high percentage of magnesium, sulfates and potassium. Dead Sea bath salts aid in the treatment of common dry skin conditions like eczema and psoriasis and is known to

Healthier Living Naturally

reduce pain and inflammation from arthritis and rheuma-tism. The high mineral content is credited with the cleansing and detoxification of the skin and with parasites. Cleopatra's favorite. **Contains: magnesium, chloride, sodium, calcium, potassium and bromide.**

- **Himalayan Pink** salt's color is a result of the trace elements in the salt. This salt includes: energy-rich **iron and 83 other natural minerals and elements.** These natural minerals are essential for human health, and can be readily absorbed through bathing. Himalayan salt has been praised for its healing benefits; and is known for stimulating circulation, soothing sore muscles, helping to reduce acid reflux, lowering blood pressure and removing toxins.

The Himalayan Salt Inhaler claims to help support rehabilitation and medical therapies of the respiratory system, including asthma. (Not FDA approved) Also for sale are salt plates that you can cook on.

Bath Salts and **Essential oils**   According to the Saltworks.us, you can use the following recipes: Mix 16 oz. of Epsom salt with 5 drops of Eucalyptus Oil and 15 drops of Lavender Oil; 16 oz. of Dead Sea salt with 20 drops of Lavender; 16 oz. of salt of Himalayan Pink Salt with 10 drops Spearmint Oil and 5 drops Rosemary Oil. (16)

All salt and essential oils should first be tried in small amounts to observe the body's reaction to oils and minerals.

"Liberty is to the collective body, what health is to every individual body. Without health no pleasure can be tasted by man; without liberty, no happiness can be enjoyed by society."

Thomas Jefferson

Healthier Living Naturally

SILVER SOL

Throughout history, silver has been used for many different things. Ancient civilizations used silver to purify the water and keep it safe from bacteria. Today, some use silver to treat a number of diseases, as well as use in health applications, such as urinary catheters and breathing tubes. The silver ion Ag is bioactive and can kill bacteria in vitro.

Not to be confused with colloidal silver, some of the many claimed uses for Silver Sol or Nano Silver (10ppm) are: Ebola, Malaria, MRSA, tumors, herpes, foot odor, warts, tuberculosis, water toxins, wounds, burns, mold, fungus, urinary tract infections and some contagious diseases such as streptococcus, staphylococcus and others.

More recent research on Silver Sol has been conducted at the following medical laboratories: University of Georgia, Kansas State, Arizona State, Brigham Young and others.

Silver Sol is considered homeopathic and should be checked for interactions with prescription medications.

RECENT RESEARCH

Silver Sol Completely Removes Malaria Parasites from the Blood of Human Subjects Infected with Malaria in an Average of Five Days: A Review of Four Randomized, Multi-Centered, Clinical Studies Performed in Africa	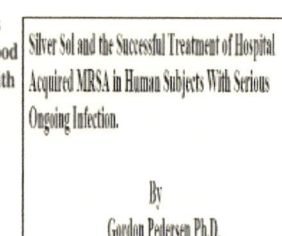	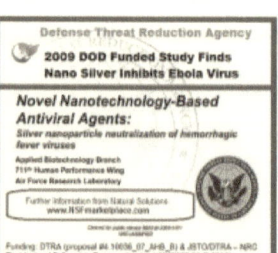

Spices and Herbs

Teas, spices and herbs have thermogenic properties and boost metabolism so you can burn more calories. They are also nutrient-dense foods that contain important vitamins, minerals, antioxidants and anti-bacterial factors to help maintain health. They stimulate digestion, cleanse the body and create energy, which are all necessary treatments for every aging part of the body, including the brain. Create a blend of your favorites and sprinkle on your food daily. (17)

ANISE is an antioxident and contains many good vitamins such as the Bs, C and A. Has a sweet taste similar to black licorice. It can calm an upset stomach and help with coughs and runny noses. It may increase milk flow in breastfeeding mothers, treat menstrual symptoms and boost libido, according to WebMD.

CALENDULA Calendula has plant antioxidants called flavonoids are often used to help ease upset stomachs, but when applied directly to the skin, may help heal burns, cuts and bruises, sore throat, as is and anti-inflammatory.

CILANTRO detoxes metals including mercury, high in vitamin K, can improves bone strength and helps the blood clot.

CINNAMON (Cassia) is an antioxidant and may help: lower blood sugar levels in people with type 2 diabetes, reduce cholesterol levels, help with gastrointestinal problems and loss of appetite, yeast infections, arthritis, boost cognitive function (i.e. test anxiety), is an E. Coli and cancer fighter, has anti-clotting properties, great source of fiber and obesity fighter. (See information on cinnamon and tumors: http://www.ncbi.nlm.nih.gov/pubmed/20653974)

CUMIN may help people with diabetes keep blood sugar levels in check, has germ-fighting properties that may prevent stomach ulcers, memory booster and is a very good source of calcium, iron and magnesium.

CLOVE is used for upset stomach and as an expectorant. Clove oil is used for diarrhea, hernia, bad breath, intestinal gas, nausea, and vomiting. It is applied directly to the mouth and gums for toothache and pain control.

DANDELION can help with liver, kidney and spleen problems; also with swelling and skin problems.

FENNEL has a similar flavor to licorice, just like anise. May help with bloating, gas, heartburn and other digestion issues.

GARLIC With garlic a new study shows it can relaxes blood vessels and increases blood flow and could reduce the risk of heart disease. It can also can ward off colds & flu.

GINGER is commonly used to treat various types of "stomach problems," including motion sickness, morning sickness, colic, upset stomach, gas, diarrhea, nausea caused by cancer treatment, nausea and vomiting after surgery, as well as loss of appetite. Other uses include pain relief from arthritis or muscle soreness, menstrual pain, upper respiratory tract infections, cough, and bronchitis. Ginger is also sometimes used for chest pain, low back pain, and stomach pain.

GINSENG American ginseng has been shown to decrease blood sugar levels in people with Type 2 diabetes, slow colorectal cancer cell growth, shorten how long colds lingers and boost immunity. Asian ginseng boost immunity, as well as improve mental health and reduce stress.

HOLY BASIL is used to treat high cholesterol. According to WebMD, other benefits included memory, upper respiratory infections, asthma, diabetes, skin, decrease swelling and pain.

LAVENDER this plant has calming and soothing qualities and can help ease stress and promote sleep. In oil form it can stop itching and swelling when used on the skin.

LICORICE root can treat coughs, asthma and heartburn. It may also help with body fat.

MILK THISTLE is an herb that may delay the growth of cancerous tumors due to its antioxidant silymarin, according to National Cancer Institute. However, the FDA has not approved its use yet.

MINT is helpful in treating a number of digestive ailments, especially irritable bowel syndrome. Peppermint oil can be effective with Irritable Bowel Syndrome. See Essential Oils.

NUTMEG fights off bacteria, fungi, and help with stomach problems and skin blemishes. Can also be a good source of fiber and have anti-inflammatory properties.

OREGANO antibacterial and *antifungal*. It has also been found to be effective against yeast-based infections like vaginitis and oral thrush.

ROSEMARY is rich in rosmarinic acid and other antioxidants, which works against **inflammation**. May help boost memory, poor circulation, water retention, dandruff and hair quality.

SAFFRON This spice can help PMS symptoms and mild to moderate depression. It's also often used to help asthma and coughs. Used also for attention deficit, memory, appetite suppressant and sleep.

SAGE is used to externally treat sprains, swelling, ulcers, and bleeding. Internally, used to treat sore throats, coughs, rheumatism, excessive menstrual bleeding, night sweats, to dry up a mother's milk when nursing was stopped, strengthening the nervous system, improving memory, and sharpening the senses.

THYME This herb is full of antioxidants which prevent cellular damage and can boost overall health and help prevent cancer, memory, inflammation, signs of aging, skin health and more.

TURMERIC "spice of life" is the main spice in curry, related to ginger; used for amlydosis, arthritis, cancer, depression, gastro, heart disease, liver disease, skin ailments (i.e. stretch marks), according to the National Institutes for Health.

*According to Dr. Jacob Teitelbaum, author of <u>Real Cause Real Cure</u>, willow bark and boswellia (Frankincense) in studies are twice as effective as ibuprofen for **arthritis**. Curamin and boswelia are more effective than some common prescriptions without the side effects.

Spiritual Health Assessment

The FICA (Faith or Belief, Importance, Community, Addressed in Care) Spiritual History Tool (Puchalski, 1996) was developed in collaboration with primary care providers as a guide for clinicians to incorporate open-ended questions regarding spirituality into a standard comprehensive history.

FICA Tool	
F – Faith, Belief, Meaning	**Religious/Religiosity** – Pertains to one's beliefs, behaviors, values, rules for conduct, and rituals associated with a specific religious tradition or denomination (O'Brien, 1999). **Spirituality** – Generally, an "individual's attitude and beliefs related to transcendence (God) or to the nonmaterial forces of life and of nature…the dimension of a person that is concerned with ultimate ends and values" and meaning (O'Brien, 1982, p. 88; Taylor, 2006).
• Do you consider yourself spiritual or religious?	
• Do you have spiritual beliefs that help you cope with stress?	
• What gives your life meaning?	
I – Importance and Influence	
• What importance does your faith or belief have in your life?	
• On a scale of 0 (not important) to 5 (very important), how would you rate the importance of faith/belief in your life?	
• Have your beliefs influenced you in how you handle stress?	
• What role do your beliefs play in your health care decision making?	
C – Community	
• Are you a part of a spiritual or religious community?	
• Is this of support to you and how?	
• Is there a group of people you really love or who are important to you?	
A – Address in Care	We have talked a lot about your spirituality and/or religious beliefs and how they may or may not be of help to you during your illness. How can your health care providers best support your spirituality?
• How would you like your health care provider to use this information about your spirituality as they care for you?	

Resource: The George Washington Institute for Spirituality and Health website, www.gwish.org

THERAPEUTIC MASSAGE

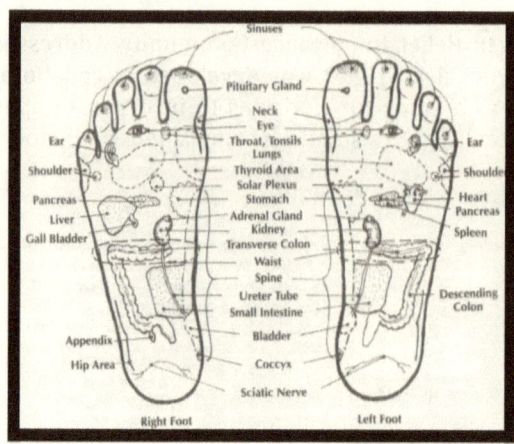

According to the Yale Journal of Medicine and Law, Reflexology is the practice of massaging, percussing and applying pressure to certain areas of the *hand, foot, or ear* to achieve a wide range of full body medical effects from pain relief to tempering aggressive children.

There are many types of massages. Here are a few:
- **Deep Tissue** is designed to relieve severe tension in the muscle and the connective tissue or fascia. This type of massage focuses on the muscles located below the surface of the top muscles.
- **Lymphatic Drainage** a technique used to gently work and stimulate the lymphatic system, to assist in reduction of localized swelling.
- **Myofascial Release** stretching the fascia and releasing bonds between connective tissue, skin, and muscles with the goal of eliminating pain, increasing range of motion and sense of balance.
- **Pediatric** is "the manual manipulation of soft tissue intended to promote health and well-being" for children and adolescents.

Healthier Living Naturally

Essential oils are often used in therapy to intensify healing.

Potential benefits: reduce the level of stress-related hormones which may increase energy and reduce stress-related diseases; improve blood circulation, blood pressure, increases the lymphatic system which eliminates lactic acid, cortical and other chemical waste; strengthen the immune system, and promote muscle relaxation. (18)

Other USEFUL INFORMATION

Did you know? 99% of the mass of the human body is made up of only six elements: oxygen, carbon, hydrogen, nitrogen, calcium, and phosphorus, and that the composition of the human body and the composition of 7 gallons of sea water are the same.

Diindolylmethane DIM - According to Memorial-Sloan Kettering, this is a compound found in vegetables including broccoli, cabbage and cauliflower. It is thought to be a superior chemo-protective compound for breast and prostate cancer. DIM demonstrated anti-proliferative effects in animals. DIM increases "good" estrogen metabolites, and simultaneously reduces the levels of "bad" estrogen metabolites.

DMSO or dimethyl sulfoxide can be used for burns, frostbite, and phantom pain.

Fruits and Vegetables Powders If you cannot get at least 7 plus servings of the fruits and vegetables that are needed each day (or half of everything we put into our mouths), there are supplements or protein powders that can help "bridge that gap."

Gelatin has collagen and is great for arthritic joints, brittle hair and nails, scoliosis, torn ligaments, weight gain, wrinkles, and is an excellent source of protein.

Healthier Living Naturally

Genetically Modified Organisms (GMO) is an organism whose genetic material has been altered using genetic engineering techniques. American farmers started growing genetically engineered (GE) crops in 1996. Many believe these altered foods could be dangerous to our health as they are designed to grow faster and resist disease. Most food is not currently labeled as such, but organic is not GMO. Dr. George Wald, Nobel laureate in physiology says this, "Recombinant DNA technology (genetic engineering) faces our society with problems unprecedented...Now whole new proteins will be transposed overnight into wholly new associations, with consequences no one can foretell...For going ahead in this direction may not only be unwise but dangerous. Potentially, it could breed new animal and plant diseases, new sources of cancer, novel epidemics." *(See: http://www.nongmoproject.org/; http://www.eatwild.com/products/index.html)*

Lymphatic System is part of the circulatory system, comprising of vessels that carry clear fluid towards the heart. Lymphatic organs are part of the immune system. Lymphoid tissue is found in lymph nodes and is associated with the digestive system such as the tonsils and other organs. The system also supports circulation and the production of lymphocytes, which includes the spleen, thymus, bone marrow, and the lymphoid tissue of the digestive system. Swollen glands are a sign the lymphatic system needs help with drainage and cleansing. Many chronically ill people have congested lymphatic systems.

*Homeopathics, Epsom Salt, cleansing teas (Green), fruits, vegetables, enzymes, vitamins (i.e. C, B complex, and Zinc), massage with essential oils and exercise can help open these channels and begin the detox process. (19)

Magnets are often marketed for different types of pain, including foot and back and from conditions such as arthritis and fibromyalgia. Various products with magnets include shoe insoles, bracelets and other jewelry, mattress pads, and bandages. Preliminary studies looked at different types of pain such as knee, hip, wrist, foot, back, and pelvic pain had mixed results. A 2007 clinical trial sponsored by the National Institutes of Health that looked at back pain in a small group, suggested a benefit from using magnets. The majority of trials, however, indicated no effect. (20)

Magnets are **not safe for people on pacemakers or have an insulin pump.

Mushrooms research supports the use of select medicinal mushrooms for their anti-inflammatory, antibacterial, antiviral, and immune-enhancing properties, including cancer care. Some good examples are: Shiitake, Enoki, Maitake, and Oyster.

Organic foods are natural and come from the earth without chemicals, pesticides or fertilizers. For better health, consider trying natural products for the home, hair, cosmetics, clothing and bedding as well.

Whole food is unprocessed and unrefined, or processed and refined as little as possible, before being consumed. They do not contain added ingredients, such as salt, carbohydrates, or fat. Examples include: unpolished grains, beans, fruits, vegetables and non-homogenized dairy products.

VITAMINS & MINERALS

As mentioned in the **Essential Minerals** section, there are **16 Essential Vitamins:** Vitamin A, Vitamin B1 (Thiamine), Vitamin B2 (Riboflavin), Vitamin B3 (Niacin), Vitamin B5 (Pantothenic Acid), Vitamin B6 (Pyridoxine), Vitamin B12 (Cobalamin), Vitamin C, Vitamin D, Vitamin E, Vitamin K, Biotin, Choline, Flavonoids and Bioflavonoids, Folic Acid, Inositol.

There are *two kinds of minerals*: **macrominerals** and **trace minerals.** The body needs organic macro minerals in larger amounts and they include: calcium, phosphorus, magnesium, sodium, potassium, chloride and sulfur. We need smaller amounts of trace minerals such as: iron, manganese, copper, iodine, zinc, cobalt and selenium. There are 91 total known minerals or elements. Experts sometimes disagree to the real number, but most agree that approximately 90 percent of Americans suffer from mineral imbalance and deficiency.

- ❖ **Calcium**...A word about too much calcium. "Calcium is an important nutrient for bone health, but new research suggests that older women who take large amounts may be at increased risk of heart disease and death... After controlling for physical activity, education, smoking, alcohol and other dietary factors, they found that women who took 1,400 milligrams or more of calcium a day had more than double the risk of death from heart disease, compared with those with intakes between 600 and 1,000 milligrams. These women also had a 49 percent higher rate of death from cardiovascular disease, and a 40 percent higher risk of death from any cause." "Extra calcium does you no good, and there is a small risk that if you take too much you might get a kidney stone," says Dr. Ethel C. Siris, director of the Toni Stabile Osteoporosis Center at Columbia University Medical Center in New York. That's because the body can only handle 600 milligrams of calcium at once. Extra calcium can build up in the bloodstream and, when excreted through kidneys in urine, it can cause a kidney stone." (21) (22).
- ❖ **Chromium** Estimates say that 90% of the population is depleted in this trace mineral. This mineral is important for blood sugar regulation and insulin function. When grain is processed, the inner endosperm, which is a source of chromium, is taken out to extend shelf life. (23)
- ❖ **Vitamin A** is important for growth and development, for the maintenance of the immune system and good vision. Vitamin A deficiency is said to sometimes be found in people with Autism, ADHD and Schizophrenia.
- ❖ **Vitamin B Complex**: thiamin (B1), riboflavin (B2), niacin (B3, also called nicotinamide or nicotinic acid amide), pantothenic acid (B5), pyridoxine (B6), biotin (B7), folic acid or folate (B9), cobalamin (B12). B vitamins are essential for growth, development, and a variety of other bodily

functions. They play a major role in the activities of enzymes, proteins that regulate chemical reactions in the body, which are important in turning food into energy and other needed substances. B vitamins are found in plant and animal food sources. People with low folate intake are at increased risk for certain types of cancer. A diet rich in vegetables and enriched grain products containing this vitamin are recommended by some experts in cancer prevention. (24) ***Folic acid supplements taken early in pregnancy (4-8 weeks) may reduce a child's risk of autism by 40 percent, according to a recent study in the Journal of the American Medical Association (25).**

❖ **Vitamin C** protects against immune system deficiencies, cardiovascular disease, prenatal health problems, eye disease, and even skin wrinkling. According to Livestrong.com, *"a **vitamin C flush** refers to the process of increasing your intake of **ascorbic acid** until your body flushes out the toxins via your stool. It is a means of determining your daily requirement of vitamin C and the dosage of ascorbic acid supplements you need to take. This is important because vitamin C is not produced or stored in humans."* *See Ascorbic Acid and cancer study (26)*

❖ **Vitamin D** Many people start to become deficient in D around middle age .The major biologic function of vitamin D is to maintain *normal blood levels of calcium* and phosphorus. Vitamin D aids in the absorption of calcium, helping to form and maintain strong bones. Recently, research also suggests that vitamin D may provide protection from osteoporosis (increase bone density), hypertension (high blood pressure), cancer, and several autoimmune diseases. You can get Vitamin D from sun exposure as well. (27) (28) **Exciting new research conducted at the Creighton University School of Medicine in Nebraska has revealed that supplementing with vitamin D and calcium can reduce your risk of cancer by an astonishing 77 percent.** This includes breast cancer, colon cancer, skin cancer and other forms of cancer. (29) (30)

WATER...Drink more!

Using a water filter with your drinking water and shower may be essential to good health. Consider testing if you have concerns, because contaminates can cause all kinds of health issues. Fluoride in water has also become concerning as of late, especially since many countries now ban it in their drinking water. To make your own alkaline water, squeeze lemon or lime into your filtered water and drink...The higher the alkaline, the better. Willard Water® has a very high alkaline pH value of 12.3.

Most people walk around dehydrated and do not intake enough water each day. According to herballegacy.com, "60-70 % of the human body contains water. The brain is composed of approximately 70% water, and the lungs are nearly 90% water. Lean muscle tissue contains approximately 75% water by weight; body fat contains 10% water and bone has 22% water. About 83% of our blood is water, which helps digest our food, transport waste, and control body temperature. Each day humans must replace at least 2.5 quarts of water, some through drinking and the rest taken by the body from the foods we eat. Beyond life giving effects, water also acts as a solvent, transporter and cleanser. All metabolic functions as well as extraction of toxins through the kidneys, the colon, the skin and the lungs rely on water. Within a 24 hour time period, about 370 gallons of blood flows through our brain and about 530 gallons of blood passes through our kidneys and liver. The human body discharges at least ½ a gallon of fluid a day and this perpetual loss of liquid must be replenished."

Bacteria, Germs, Pathogens, Microbes, Viruses, Parasites and their eggs are all known as microorganisms. These minute living organisms, germs and viruses cause Water Borne Diseases. Infection commonly results during bathing, washing, drinking, in the preparation of food, or the consumption of food from these microorganisms.

Chlorine "Health officials are concerned with the chlorinating by-products, also known as "chlorinated hydrocarbons" or trihalomethanes (THM's). Most THM's are formed in drinking water when chlorine reacts with naturally occurring substances such as decomposing plant and animal materials. **Risks for certain types of cancer are now being correlated to the consumption of chlorinated drinking water.** The President's Council on Environmental Quality states that "there is increased evidence for an association between rectal, colon and bladder cancer and the consumption of chlorinated drinking water." Suspected carcinogens make the human body more vulnerable through repeated ingestion and research indicates the incidence of cancer is 44% higher among those using chlorinated water." (31)

Plastic Water Bottles are made from polyethylene terephthalate. When heated, the material releases the chemicals antimony, which is considered a carcinogen by the International Agency for Research on Cancer, and bisphenol A which is commonly called a BPA. More attention should be given to other drinks packaged with polyethylene terephthalate plastic, such as milk, coffee and acidic juice as well.

Ionized Water is drinking water that has undergone a process known as ionization. This process segregates the acid and alkaline content found in H2O. The water goes through the electrolysis process, taking advantage of the naturally occurring electric charge found within magnesium and calcium ions. When successfully ionized, it is said that this type of drinking water can help enhance the ability of the blood to carry oxygen and also assist in neutralizing free radicals in the bloodstream. **Distilled Water** is water that is purified of contaminants through the distillation process. Water is brought to a boil and converted to steam. The steam flows through cooling tubes and condenses back into pure water. This is different than filtering water. This process is supposed to remove potentially harmful organisms and chemicals.

Looking for a clean, natural spring near you?
Go to http://www.findaspring.com.

Did you know? A 2% drop in body water can trigger: fuzzy short-term memory, trouble with basic math and difficulty focusing on the computer screen or a printed page. Caffeine has a diuretic effect, pulling water out of cells and the body, further promoting dehydration. ***To replace the water lost from soft drinks, one needs to consume 8-12 glasses for every glass of soda consumed.** *(www.pathmed.com)

"X"TRA "Y"EAST AND "D"ISEASES

Yeast is a common infection caused by a fungus* known as Candida albicans, which can spread to other parts of the body via the bloodstream if not taken care of immediately. The yeast attaches itself to the walls of the intestines and can make tiny perforations into the wall to allow toxins from the yeast to enter. The toxins are then pumped all over the body.

*Fungus is any member of a kingdom of organisms (Fungi) that lack chlorophyll, leaves, true stems, and roots, reproduce by spores, and live as parasites. The group includes molds, mildews, rusts, yeasts, and mushrooms.

Dr. William Shaw, founder of The Great Plains Laboratory, Inc. has this to say about yeast..."Elevation of yeast metabolites such as tartaric acid and arabinose are found in many of the same disorders and are even more common in **autism, SLE, Alzheimer's disease, fibromyalgia, attention deficit hyperactivity, and Chronic Fatigue Syndrome**. The arabinose may interfere with gluconeogenesis and also may through pentosidine formation significantly alter protein structure, transport, solubility, and enzymatic activity as well as triggering autoimmune reactions to the modified proteins. The finding of pentosidine in the neurofibrillary tangles of Alzheimer's brains and its absence from normal areas of the brain may indicate a direct role of a yeast byproduct in accelerating the normal aging process. Tartaric acid from yeast overgrowth has a direct toxic effect on muscles and is an inhibitor of a key Krebs cycle enzyme that supplies raw materials for gluconeogenesis and offers an explanation for many of the symptoms of fibromyalgia."
(32)

Did You Know? **Apple cider vinegar** is rich in natural enzymes and is said to regulate the presence of candida in the body. It helps encourage the growth of healthy bacteria, which in turn minimizes the overgrowth of candida. Apple cider vinegar also helps balance your body's pH level. In **"Cancer is a Fungus"** by Dr. T. Simoncini, Candida and fungus is explained in terms of its opportunistic behavior, its similar genetic structure to cancer, its constant presence in cancer tumors and the phenomenon of metastasis. Detoxing is extremely important for getting rid of these traveling toxins. *Flor Essence®* would be an example of a detoxifier and Dr. Simoncini uses sodium bicarbonate or baking soda.

Appendix

MY PERSONAL HEALTH AND WELLNESS ASSESSMENT

TODAY'S DATE: _____

The benefits of taking a health and wellness assessment include:

- Creates a baseline for healthy wellbeing
- Creates a basis for potential lifestyles changes
- Prepares and encourages healthy weight and life-style
- Identifies needs and deficiencies in diet and nutrition
- Develops a personal results-oriented program

Using the scale 1 to 10 rate the following:

1. Physical Health _____

2. Mental Health _____

3. Spiritual Health _____

Complete the following:

1. My Body Mass Index (BMI) _____

2. My weight _____

3. My Blood Pressure _____

4. My Blood Sugar _____

5. My Cholesterol Level _____

6. My Maximum Heart Rate _____

7. My Minimum Heart Rate _____

MY HEALTH PLAN

IDENTIFY:

FIVE GOALS FOR MYSELF IN THE NEXT YEAR:

1. _____

2. _____

3. _____

4. _____

5. _____

THREE STEPS TO BETTER HEALTH THAT I CAN TAKE STARTING TODAY:

1. _____

2. _____

3. _____

Where to Begin...

After reading this handbook, some readers might be confused where to begin. There is so much information and it can be overwhelming. You may have to do a little at a time, but that is okay. Whatever you do, begin to create healthy habits. Changes won't take place unless you do these things DAILY. Consider journaling and record your health plan so that you can see your goals and results.

Here are some suggestions to get started TODAY:

1. Get a physical.
2. Start eating healthier—MORE FRUITS AND VEGETABLES.
3. Begin to eliminate junk food and sweets as much as possible.
4. Cut out soda, drink organic teas, filtered water with lemon instead.
5. Consider smaller servings of meat and dairy. See *Forks over Knives*.
6. Neutralize your pH with apple cider vinegar.
7. Make a daily smoothie with fruits, vegetables, perhaps a protein powder AND an omega-3 source.
8. Every day take a strong probiotic for the gut.
9. Get a good multi vitamin. Consider other super food supplements.
10. Exercise, however that looks like for you.
11. Get a massage or visit the chiropractor to help release toxins.
12. Take salt baths or soaks. Consider essential oils.
13. Do a detox regimen to get rid of toxins such as Flor Essence.
14. Get more sleep and try to reduce stress.
15. Use spices in your food daily.
16. Introduce coconut and olive oil into your diet.
17. Try to buy organic and non-GMO food and products.
18. Complete Dr. Braverman's Age Print and Brain Quiz. (Brain Health)
19. Visit your local health food and whole food store.
20. Begin working on your spiritual, physical and mental health today!

OTHER THOUGHTS

_____

_____

_____

_____

_____

_____

_____

_____

_____

_____

_____

_____

_____

Notes

1. *"Welcome to the China-Cornell-Oxford Project." Welcome to the China-Cornell-Oxford Project. N.p., n.d. Web. 23 Feb. 2013

2. "Electrodermal Screening." YouTube. YouTube, 28 Jan. 2010. Web. 21 Feb. 2013. "Compass." ZYTO. N.p., n.d. Web. 21 Feb. 2013.

3. "Apple Cider Vinegar Uses, Benefits, Claims." WebMD. WebMD, n.d. Web. 21 Feb. 2013.

4. "Amino Acids: MedlinePlus Medical Encyclopedia." U.S National Library of Medicine. U.S. National Library of Medicine, n.d. Web. 26 Feb. 2013.

5. Breathing Slower and Less: The Greatest Health Discovery Ever?" Breathing Slower and Less The Greatest Health Discovery Ever? N.p., n.d. Web. 24 Feb. 2013.

6. Source: "Why Detox? â"Shedding Light on Detoxification." Why Detox. N.p., n.d. Web. 23 Feb. 2013.

7. Centers for Disease Control and Prevention. Centers for Disease Control and Prevention, 01 Feb. 2012. Web. 23 Feb. 2013.

8. "Enzyme." Wikipedia. Wikimedia Foundation, 26 Feb. 2013. Web. 04 Mar. 2013.

9. Velasquez-manoff, Moises. "OPINION; What Really Causes Celiac Disease?" The New York Times. The New York Times, 24 Feb. 2013. Web. 25 Feb. 2013.

10. "Think Twice: How the Gut's "Second Brain" Influences Mood and Well-Being: Scientific American. N.p., n.d. Web. 07 Mar. 2013.

11. "Magnesium." â" Health Professional Fact Sheet. N.p., n.d. Web. 02 Mar. 2013.

12. "Folk Medicine." Randomhouse.com. N.p., n.d. Web. 14 Mar. 2013.

13. "Potassium in Diet: MedlinePlus Medical Encyclopedia." U.S National Library of Medicine. U.S. National Library of Medicine, n.d. Web. 02 Mar. 2013.

14. Aborn, Shana. "Probiotics: Good for More Than Digestion." Health Radar 3 (Apr. 2013): 1-2. Print.

15. "FDA Warns Azithromycin "Z-pack" Antibiotics Could Lead to Deadly Heart Rhythms for Some." CBSNews. CBS Interactive, n.d. Web. 13 Mar. 2013

Healthier Living Naturally

16. "Sea Salt Information." Sea Salts & Bath Salts. N.p., n.d. Web. 22 Feb. 2013

17. Feature, Elizabeth M. Ward, MS, RDWebMD. "Spices & Herbs Health Benefits and Adding Spices to Foods." WebMD. WebMD, n.d. Web. 02 Mar. 2013.

18. "The Mechanisms of Massage and Effects on Performance, Muscle Recovery and Injury Prevention." Latest TOC RSS. N.p., n.d. Web. 23 Feb. 2013.

19. "How to Do a Lymph Cleansing Diet." LIVESTRONG.COM. N.p., n.d. Web. 07 Mar. 2013

20. "Magnets for Pain." Home Page. N.p., n.d. Web. 14 Mar. 2013. <http://nccam.nih.gov/health/magnet/magnetsforpain.htm>.

21. Neighmond, Patti. "Too Much Calcium Could Cause Kidney, Heart Problems, Researchers Say." NPR. NPR, 13 Aug. 2012. Web. 23 Feb. 2013.

22. "Dangers of Too Much Calcium." Well Dangers of Too Much Calcium Comments. N.p., n.d. Web. 23 Feb. 2013.

23. "Chromium." Dietary Supplement Fact Sheet: â🔲" Health Professional Fact Sheet. N.p., n.d. Web. 23 Feb. 2013.

24. "Vitamin B Complex." Vitamin B Complex. N.p., n.d. Web. 23 Feb. 2013.

25. "Folic Acid Supplements Early in Pregnancy May Reduce Child🔲™s Risk of Autism by 40 Percent." Bjrklund Nutrition. N.p., n.d. Web. 16 Mar. 2013.

26. http://www.pnas.org/content/102/38/13604.full

27. Mayo Clinic. Mayo Foundation for Medical Education and Research, 01 Sept. 2012. Web. 23 Feb. 2013.

28. "Vitamins and Minerals: How Much Do You Need?" WebMD. WebMD, n.d. Web. 02 Mar. 2013

29. "New Research Shows Vitamin D Slashes Risk of Cancers by 77 Percent; Cancer Industry Refuses to Support Cancer Prevention." Natural News. N.p., n.d. Web. 30 Apr. 2013.

30. "The Periodic Table of Vitamins." Daily Burn Blog The Periodic Table of Vitamins Comments. N.p., n.d. Web. 02 Mar. 2013.

31. Source: "Chlorine's Adverse Health Effects." Chlorine's Adverse Health Effects. N.p., n.d. Web. 23 Feb. 2013.

32. http://www.greatplainslaboratory.com/home/eng/candida.asp

www.ingramcontent.com/pod-product-compliance
Lightning Source LLC
Chambersburg PA
CBHW020357290526
45785CB00005B/2328